DIABETES DIET
COOKBOOK
AFTER 50

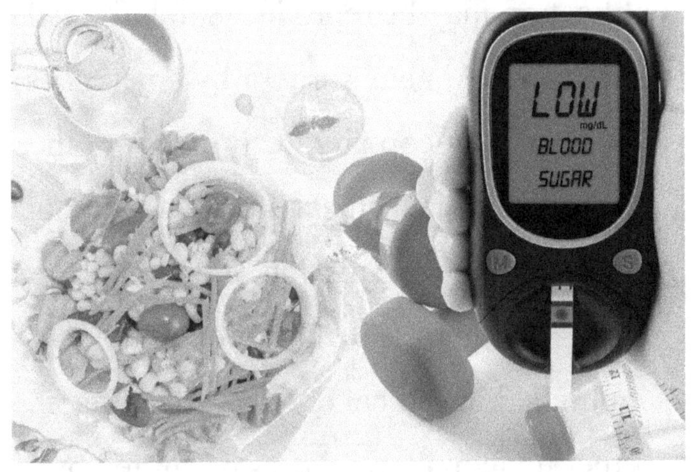

The recipes are quick and easy to prepare.

Keri K. Huey

TABLE OF CONTENTS

INTRODUCTION

Thomas was in his late fifties and had been diabetic for more than a decade. Despite his best efforts, he suffered with variable blood sugar levels and had encountered various difficulties over the years. Thomas was unhappy and weary of fighting his health all the time.

While wandering at a neighborhood bookshop one day, Thomas came upon a book named "The Diabetes Diet Cookbook After 50." He chose to buy the cookbook since it promised a better living. He had no idea that such a simple action would affect his life forever.

As Thomas went through the cookbook's pages, he was astounded by the range of tasty and healthy meals designed exclusively for diabetics. The book stressed the significance of eating a well-balanced diet rich in natural foods, lean proteins, and carbs with a low glycemic index. It also gave useful advice on portion management and mindful eating.

Thomas started experimenting with the recipes, eager to give it a go. He began to spend more time in the kitchen, experimenting with different tastes and ingredients. He substituted healthful meals like fresh fruits, vegetables, and entire grains for processed foods and sugary snacks. Thomas learned that cooking might be a therapeutic pastime, enabling him to take positive control of his health.

Thomas began to notice dramatic improvements in only a few weeks. His energy levels increased, and he no longer suffered from the chronic weariness that had plagued him for years. His blood sugar levels normalized, lowering the requirement for insulin injections on a regular basis. During his routine check-up, his doctor was astounded by the good change.

Thomas grew more committed to his newfound lifestyle as a result of his success. He began to include fitness in his daily routine, going for lengthy walks in the park and doing yoga for flexibility and relaxation. He also joined a local diabetic support group, where he found comfort in interacting with people who had gone through similar things.

Thomas became healthier and happy with each passing day. The cookbook had not only given him excellent recipes, but it had also given him a thorough grasp of healthy nutrition and self-care. He became a diabetes awareness champion, sharing his story with others and pushing them to take responsibility of their own health.

Thomas celebrated his 60th birthday a year later with fresh vigour. He was characterized no longer by his diabetes, but by his perseverance and resolve to live a meaningful life. He proceeded to experiment with new recipes, tailoring them to his tastes and introducing a diverse variety of flavors and ingredients into his meals.

Thomas' tale went across the neighborhood, motivating others to choose a better lifestyle. He became a beacon of hope for those living with diabetes, demonstrating that it was possible to flourish even in the face of hardship with the correct tools and mentality.

Thomas eventually decided to publish his own cookbook, offering his own experiences, recipes, and diabetes management suggestions. He aspired to provide people with the information and encouragement they needed to make meaningful life changes.

Thomas' diabetes path has changed from one of struggle and frustration to one of optimism and victory. He not only found the way to improved health, but also rekindled his enthusiasm for life, thanks to the magic of the diabetic diet cookbook.

As a result, Thomas' experience serves as a reminder that it is never too late to take charge of our health. No of our age or circumstances, we can overcome any hurdle and enjoy a full, happy life with dedication, a supportive community, and the correct resources.

WHAT IS DIABETES ?

Diabetes is a long-term medical disorder defined by excessive blood sugar (glucose) levels. It happens when the body does not create enough insulin or when the cells do not react adequately to the insulin that is produced. Insulin is a hormone that controls glucose uptake and use by cells in the body.

Diabetes is classified into two types: type 1 and type 2.

Type 1 diabetes, also known as insulin-dependent diabetes or juvenile-onset diabetes, often manifests itself during childhood or adolescence. The body's immune system assaults and kills insulin-producing cells in the pancreas in this kind. As a consequence, the body is unable to manufacture insulin, resulting in hyperglycemia. Type 1 diabetes requires daily insulin injections or the use of an insulin pump to keep blood sugar levels under control.

Type 2 diabetes, commonly known as non-insulin-dependent diabetes or adult-onset diabetes, is more frequent and occurs later in life. The body may create insulin in this case, but either not enough or the cells develop resistant to its effects. Obesity, sedentary lifestyle, family history, and certain ethnic origins are all risk factors for type 2 diabetes. Initially, dietary and activity changes may suffice to treat type 2 diabetes. Some people, however, may need oral drugs or insulin injections to keep their blood sugar levels under control.

Both kinds of diabetes may induce high blood sugar levels, which can lead to a variety of health concerns if not managed. Cardiovascular difficulties, nerve damage (neuropathy), kidney illness (nephropathy), eye damage (retinopathy), foot problems, and an increased risk of infections are among the consequences.

Diabetes management is regularly checking blood sugar levels, eating a nutritious diet, exercising regularly, and taking prescription drugs or insulin as instructed by a healthcare expert. Individuals with diabetes must collaborate closely with their healthcare team to design a specific treatment plan and make lifestyle changes in order to maintain their blood sugar levels within a target range. Furthermore, diabetes self-care education and symptom awareness are critical for early identification and adequate treatment.

WHAT IS DIABETES DIET

A diabetes diet, also known as medical nutrition treatment or MNT, is a manner of eating that assists diabetics in managing their blood sugar levels and general health. A diabetic diet's key aims are to control blood glucose levels, maintain a healthy weight, and avoid or manage diabetes complications.

Here are some major diabetic diet principles:

1. Carbohydrate Counting: Carbohydrates have the greatest influence on blood glucose levels. Controlling and monitoring carbohydrate consumption is critical in diabetes management. Typically, the total quantity of carbs ingested throughout the day is split between equally spaced meals and snacks. Carbohydrate counting allows people to match the quantity of carbs they ingest to their insulin dosages or oral medicines.

2. Portion Control: Portion control is vital for calorie management, weight management, and avoiding blood sugar spikes. Balanced carbohydrate, protein, and fat intake at each meal may help manage blood sugar levels and offer appropriate nutrients.

3. Select Healthy carbs: Not all carbs are the same. It is critical to prioritize the consumption of nutritious carbs such as whole grains, fruits, vegetables, and legumes. These meals are high in fiber, which slows glucose absorption into the circulation and results in more stable blood sugar levels.

4. Limit Sugary Foods and Beverages: Foods and beverages rich in added sugars may trigger blood sugar increases. It is best to limit your intake of sugary drinks, candies, desserts, and processed foods. Artificial sweeteners may be used as a substitute, although moderation is still advised.

5. Include Lean Proteins: Proteins are important for controlling blood sugar levels and promoting fullness. Select lean protein sources such as chicken, fish, tofu, lentils, and low-fat dairy products. Avoid fried and high-fat protein sources.

6. Healthy Fats: Include avocados, nuts, seeds, and olive oil in your diet as sources of healthy fats. These fats may promote heart health and give you a sense of fullness. However, it is important to regulate fat consumption in order to control calorie consumption and maintain a healthy weight.

7. Meal time: Meal time consistency is good for diabetes control. Eating meals and snacks at regular intervals throughout the day may help manage blood sugar levels and avoid extreme variations.

8. Stay Hydrated: Water is the finest hydration option. Reduce your intake of sugary drinks and replace them with water, unsweetened tea, or infused water.

It is crucial to note that each person's dietary requirements will differ depending on variables such as age, weight, exercise level, medicines, and general health. A registered dietitian or a healthcare practitioner who specializes in diabetic nutrition may give individualized direction and help in designing an optimal meal plan suited to individual requirements and tastes.

A diabetic diet is about making educated and balanced choices to promote optimum blood sugar management and general well-being, not about severe restriction or avoiding whole food categories.

WHY IS IT IMPORTANT FOR INDIVIDUAL OVER 50's

Diabetes becomes especially significant beyond the age of 50 since this is when the chance of acquiring the illness tends to grow. Here are a few reasons why diabetes control is so important for those in their 50s and beyond:

1. Increased Risk: The likelihood of having type 2 diabetes increases with age. People's bodies may become less effective at utilising insulin as they age, and they may also be more likely to be overweight or have other risk factors for diabetes. As a result, people in their 50s and beyond are more likely to acquire diabetes than those in younger age groups.

2. issues: Uncontrolled diabetes may lead to a variety of health issues that can have a major effect on overall well-being. Heart disease, stroke, renal disease, nerve damage, vision issues, and foot troubles are some of these consequences. People may already be at a greater risk for these problems as they age, and having diabetes raises the probability even more. Diabetes therapy may help lower the risk and development of these problems.

3. Pre-existing Health disorders: People in their 50s and beyond are more likely to have pre-existing health disorders such as high blood pressure, high cholesterol levels, and obesity. Diabetes and these disorders often coexist and may increase its impact on the body. Effective diabetes treatment may enhance overall health and the management of other concomitant health concerns.

4. Quality of Life: Diabetes may have a negative influence on a person's quality of life, particularly as they become older. Uncontrolled diabetes may induce tiredness, frequent urination, excessive thirst, and hazy eyesight, all of which can interfere with everyday activities and diminish overall well-being. Individuals may increase their energy levels, cognitive function, and general quality of life by correctly regulating their blood sugar levels.

5. Complication Prevention: While it is critical to treat current diabetes, it is also critical to avoid the development of diabetes in the first place. Adopting a healthy lifestyle, keeping a balanced diet, participating in regular physical exercise, and controlling weight may dramatically lower the risk of getting diabetes in those in their 50s and beyond. Regular tests and check-ups may aid in the early detection of diabetic symptoms, allowing for appropriate intervention.

TIPS FOR FOLLOWING THE DIABETES DIET

1. Seek the advice of a certified dietician or a healthcare professional: Consult a healthcare practitioner or a qualified dietician who specializes in diabetes care for advice. They may provide tailored suggestions based on your unique requirements, taking into account aspects such as blood sugar levels, weight, exercise level, and general health.

2. Keep track of your carbohydrate intake: Carbohydrates have the greatest influence on blood sugar levels. Learn to recognize and monitor dietary carbohydrate content. Consume complex carbs such as whole grains, legumes, fruits, and vegetables while avoiding processed carbohydrates and sugary meals.

3. meal control: Pay attention to meal proportions to avoid overeating and efficiently regulate blood sugar levels. To determine suitable serving amounts, use measuring cups, a food scale, or visual cues (for example, a deck of cards for protein).

4. use healthy fats: Instead of saturated and trans fats, use healthy fats such as avocados, nuts, seeds, and olive oil. Healthy fats may aid with insulin sensitivity and heart health.

5. Include lean proteins: Include lean protein sources in your meals such as skinless chicken, fish, tofu, lentils, and low-fat dairy products. Protein improves fullness and helps to normalize blood sugar levels.

6. Eat regular meals and snacks: Establish a regimen of regular meals and snacks to keep blood sugar levels steady throughout the day. To avoid blood sugar spikes or decreases, avoid large pauses between meals.

7. Fiber-rich foods: Consume fiber-rich meals to help manage blood sugar levels and enhance digestive health. Choose whole grains, veggies, fruits, legumes, and nuts instead.

8. Avoid or reduce your use of sugary beverages such as soda, sweetened juices, and energy drinks. These may result in fast blood sugar increases.

9. remain hydrated: To remain hydrated, drink lots of water throughout the day. Water is the greatest beverage option for those with diabetes.

10. frequent physical exercise: Follow your healthcare professional's recommendations for frequent physical activity. Exercise may aid with insulin sensitivity, weight management, and general well-being.

11. Regularly check your blood sugar levels using a glucose meter or a continuous glucose monitoring device. This helps you to make necessary changes to your diet and lifestyle.

12. consume alcohol in moderation and with care: If you want to consume alcohol, do it in moderation and with caution. Alcohol may induce blood sugar swings and may interfere with diabetic medications.

CHAPTER 1

DELICIOUS BREAKFAST RECIPES

Veggie Omelette

Ingredients:

- 2 large eggs
- 2 tablespoons of diced bell peppers (any color you prefer)
- 2 tablespoons of diced onions
- 2 tablespoons of diced tomatoes
- 2 tablespoons of chopped spinach
- 2 tablespoons of shredded cheddar cheese
- Salt and pepper to taste
- 1 teaspoon of olive oil

Instructions:

1. Whisk the eggs in a mixing basin until completely combined. Season with salt and pepper to your liking.

2. In a nonstick skillet over medium heat, heat the olive oil.

3. Add the diced bell peppers and onions to the pan and cook for 2-3 minutes, or until tender.

4. Sauté the diced tomatoes and chopped spinach in the pan for another 1-2 minutes, or until the spinach wilts slightly.

5. Make sure the beaten eggs cover the whole surface of the sautéed veggies in the pan.

6. Allow the omelette to cook for a few minutes, or until the edges begin to solidify.

7. Evenly distribute the shredded cheddar cheese over the omelette.

8. Fold one side of the omelette carefully over the filling to form a half-moon shape.

9. Cook for another minute or two, or until the cheese melts and the omelette is done.

10. Place the vegetarian omelette on a platter and serve immediately.

Berry Yogurt Parfait

Ingredients:

- 1 cup of Greek yogurt
- 1 cup of mixed berries (such as strawberries, blueberries, raspberries)
- 1/4 cup of granola
- 1 tablespoon of honey (optional)
- Fresh mint leaves for garnish (optional)

Instructions:

1. Begin by placing 1/4 cup Greek yogurt at the bottom of a glass or dish.

2. On top of the yogurt, put a layer of mixed berries.

3. A spoonful of granola should be sprinkled over the fruit.

4. Layer another 1/4 cup yogurt, additional berries, and another tablespoon granola on top.

5. Finally, add a layer of yogurt on top.

6. If desired, drizzle honey over the top layer to add sweetness.

7. Garnish with fresh mint leaves for a burst of flavor.

8. Serve right away and enjoy!

Avocado Toast with Poached Eggs

Ingredients:

- 2 slices of whole-grain bread
- 1 ripe avocado
- 2 large eggs
- Salt and pepper to taste
- Optional toppings: sliced cherry tomatoes, feta cheese, red pepper flakes, fresh herbs

Instructions:

1. Toast the whole-grain bread pieces to your preferred crispiness.

2. While the bread toasts, cut the ripe avocado in half, remove the pit, and scoop out the meat.

3. With a fork, mash the avocado until it reaches the required consistency. You have the option of leaving it somewhat lumpy or smooth.

4. Season the mashed avocado to taste with salt and pepper.

5. Once the bread has been toasted, evenly sprinkle the mashed avocado on each piece.

6. Bring water to a simmer in a medium-sized pot. To help the eggs remain intact when poaching, add a drop of vinegar.

7. One egg should be cracked into a small cup or ramekin.

8. Using a spoon, create a gently vortex in the boiling water, then delicately slip the egg into the middle of the whirlpool.

9. Rep the procedure with the second egg.

10. Allow the eggs to poach for 3-4 minutes for a soft yolk, or longer for a firmer yolk.

11. While the eggs are poaching, top your avocado toast with optional toppings like sliced cherry tomatoes, crumbled feta cheese, red pepper flakes, or fresh herbs.

12. When the eggs are done to your satisfaction, gently take them from the water with a slotted spoon and allow any extra water to drain.

13. On each piece of avocado toast, place one poached egg.

14. Season with salt and pepper to taste, then top with any preferred toppings.

15. Serve right away and enjoy!

Banana Pancakes

Ingredients:

- 1 ripe banana
- 2 eggs
- 1/4 cup of whole wheat flour or oat flour
- 1/2 teaspoon of baking powder
- 1/2 teaspoon of vanilla extract
- Optional toppings: fresh berries, sliced bananas, maple syrup, nuts, or yogurt

Instructions:

1. Mash the ripe banana with a fork in a mixing dish until smooth.
2. Whisk together the eggs and the mashed banana until fully mixed.
3. To the banana and egg mixture, add the whole wheat flour or oat flour, baking powder, and vanilla extract. Stir until all of the ingredients are combined and a batter forms.

4. Melt butter in a nonstick pan or griddle over medium heat.

5. Grease the skillet lightly with cooking spray or a little quantity of oil.

6. For each pancake, spoon roughly 1/4 cup of the pancake mixture onto the skillet.

7. Cook for 2-3 minutes, or until bubbles appear on the pancake's surface.

8. Cook the pancake for a further 1-2 minutes, or until golden brown.

9. Repeat with the remaining batter, adjusting the heat as required to avoid burning.

10. Stack the banana pancakes on a dish and top with your favorite toppings, such as fresh berries, sliced bananas, maple syrup, almonds, or yogurt.

11. Serve right away and enjoy!

Spinach and Feta Egg Muffins

Ingredients:

- 6 large eggs
- 1 cup of fresh spinach, chopped
- 1/4 cup of crumbled feta cheese
- 1/4 cup of diced bell peppers
- 1/4 cup of diced onions
- Salt and pepper to taste
- Optional add-ins: chopped tomatoes, mushrooms, cooked bacon, or herbs of your choice

Instructions:

1. Preheat your oven to 350°F (175°C) and gently oil or line a muffin tray with paper liners.
2. In a mixing bowl, whisk the eggs until thoroughly combined. Season with salt and pepper to taste.
3. Whisk in the chopped spinach, crumbled feta cheese, diced bell peppers, and diced

onions. To blend, mix everything together well.

4. If desired, add alternative ingredients like as diced tomatoes, mushrooms, cooked bacon, or herbs of your choosing. Stir to combine.

5. Fill each muffin cup approximately 3/4 full with the egg mixture.

6. Bake for 18-20 minutes, or until the egg muffins are firm and slightly browned on top.

7. Remove from the oven and set aside to cool for a few minutes.

8. Remove the egg muffins from the muffin tray and serve.

9.

10. These spinach and feta egg muffins make an excellent make-ahead breakfast. You may keep them in the refrigerator for up to 3-4 days in an airtight container.

Before serving, just reheat in the microwave or oven.

Overnight Chia Pudding

Ingredients:

- 1/4 cup of chia seeds
- 1 cup of unsweetened almond milk (or any other milk of your choice)
- 1 tablespoon of maple syrup or honey
- 1/2 teaspoon of vanilla extract
- Optional toppings: fresh berries, sliced bananas, chopped nuts, shredded coconut, or a drizzle of nut

Instructions:

1. Combine the chia seeds, unsweetened almond milk, maple syrup or honey, and vanilla essence in a dish or container. Stir well to ensure that the chia seeds are uniformly dispersed.

2. Refrigerate the dish or jar overnight or for at least 4 hours to enable the chia seeds to absorb the liquid and thicken.

3. Give the chia pudding a thorough stir after it has set and achieved the desired consistency.

4. Toppings such as fresh berries, sliced bananas, chopped almonds, shredded coconut, or a drizzle of nut butter may be added to the chia pudding in bowls or jars.

5. Enjoy your creamy, nutrient-dense chia pudding!

6.

7. This overnight chia pudding is not only tasty, but it's also high in fiber, omega-3 fatty acids, and antioxidants from the chia seeds. It's a filling and nutritious breakfast alternative that you can prepared ahead of time.

Peanut Butter Banana Smoothie

Ingredients:

- 1 ripe banana
- 2 tablespoons of peanut butter (smooth or crunchy)
- 1 cup of unsweetened almond milk (or any other milk of your choice)
- 1/2 cup of Greek yogurt (optional for added creaminess)
- 1 tablespoon of honey or maple syrup (optional for added sweetness)
- 1/2 teaspoon of vanilla extract
- A handful of ice cubes

Instructions:

1. Peel the ripe banana and cut it into slices.
2. In a blender, add the banana chunks, peanut butter, almond milk, Greek yogurt (if using), honey or maple syrup (if used), vanilla extract, and ice cubes.

3. Blend on high until all of the ingredients are fully incorporated and the smoothie has a smooth and creamy smoothness.

4. If necessary, pause to scrape down the sides of the blender, then mix briefly again.

5. If desired, taste the smoothie and modify the sweetness or peanut butter flavor.

6. Pour the smoothie into a glass and serve immediately.

Blueberry Oatmeal Muffins

Ingredients:

- 1 cup of rolled oats
- 1 cup of whole wheat flour
- 1/4 cup of honey or maple syrup
- 1 teaspoon of baking powder
- 1/2 teaspoon of baking soda
- 1/4 teaspoon of salt

- 1 cup of unsweetened almond milk (or any other milk of your choice)
- 1/4 cup of unsweetened applesauce
- 1 teaspoon of vanilla extract
- 1 cup of fresh or frozen blueberries

Instructions:

1. Preheat the oven to 350°F (175°C) and prepare a muffin pan with paper liners.
2. Combine the rolled oats, whole wheat flour, baking powder, baking soda, and salt in a mixing dish. To combine the dry ingredients, whisk them together well.
3. Whisk together the honey or maple syrup, almond milk, unsweetened applesauce, and vanilla extract in a separate dish.
4. Mix the wet ingredients into the dry ingredients until just mixed. Overmixing the batter may result in denser muffins.
5. Fold in the blueberries gently, taking care not to bruise them.

6. Divide the mixture equally among the muffin cups, filling them approximately two-thirds full.

7. Bake for 18-20 minutes, or until a toothpick inserted in the middle of a muffin comes out clean.

8. Remove from the oven and rest for a few minutes in the pan before transferring to a wire rack to cool entirely.

9. These blueberry oatmeal muffins are a filling and flavorful morning alternative. They're high in fiber from the oats and whole wheat flour, antioxidants from the blueberries, and natural sweetness from honey or maple syrup.

CHAPTER 2

Lunch recipes

Quinoa Salad with Roasted Vegetables

Ingredients:

- 1 cup quinoa
- 2 cups water or vegetable broth
- 1 red bell pepper, sliced
- 1 zucchini, sliced
- 1 yellow squash, sliced
- 1 red onion, sliced
- 2 tablespoons olive oil
- 1 teaspoon dried oregano
- Salt and pepper to taste
- Juice of 1 lemon
- 2 tablespoons chopped fresh parsley
- Optional: crumbled feta cheese or toasted almonds for garnish

Instructions:

1. Preheat the oven to 400 degrees Fahrenheit (200 degrees Celsius).

2. Drain the quinoa after rinsing it in cold water. Bring the water or vegetable broth to a boil in a saucepan. Reduce the heat to low, cover, and simmer for 15-20 minutes, or until the quinoa is tender and the liquid has been absorbed.

3. Meanwhile, line a baking sheet with sliced bell pepper, zucchini, yellow squash, and red onion. Drizzle with olive oil and season with salt and pepper to taste. Toss to evenly coat the veggies.

4. Roast the veggies for 20-25 minutes, or until soft and slightly caramelized, in a preheated oven.

5. Combine the cooked quinoa and roasted veggies in a large mixing basin. Squeeze the lemon juice over the salad and gently stir.

6. Garnish with fresh parsley and crumbled feta cheese or roasted almonds, if preferred.

7. As a delightful and healthy lunch alternative, serve warm or cold.

Chickpea Avocado Wrap

Ingredients:

- 1 can chickpeas, drained and rinsed
- 1 ripe avocado, mashed
- 1 tablespoon lemon juice
- 2 tablespoons Greek yogurt
- 1/4 teaspoon cumin
- Salt and pepper to taste
- 4 whole wheat tortillas
- Sliced cucumbers, tomatoes, and lettuce for filling
- Optional: hummus or tahini sauce for spreading

Instructions:

1. Combine the chickpeas, mashed avocado, lemon juice, Greek yogurt, cumin, salt, and pepper in a mixing bowl. With a fork, mash the ingredients until thoroughly incorporated but still somewhat chunky.

2. Lay out the whole wheat tortillas and, if preferred, put a small coating of hummus or tahini sauce on each tortilla.

3. Distribute the chickpea avocado mixture equally among the tortillas, focusing on the center of each.

4. Top with cucumber, tomato, and lettuce slices.

5. Fold the tortilla's edges inside, then roll it up firmly from the bottom to form a wrap.

6. If preferred, cut the wraps in half and serve immediately, or pack them for a portable lunch alternative.

Grilled Chicken Salad with Balsamic Vinaigrette

Ingredients:

- 2 boneless, skinless chicken breasts
- Salt and pepper to taste
- 8 cups mixed salad greens
- 1 cup cherry tomatoes, halved
- 1/2 cup sliced red onions
- 1/4 cup crumbled feta cheese
- 1/4 cup chopped walnuts
- For the Balsamic Vinaigrette:
- 1/4 cup balsamic vinegar
- 2 tablespoons extra-virgin olive oil
- 1 tablespoon Dijon mustard
- 1 teaspoon honey
- Salt and pepper to taste

Instructions:

1. Preheat the grill or grill pan over medium-high heat.

2. Season both sides of the chicken breasts with salt and pepper.

3. Grill the chicken breasts for 6-8 minutes each side, or until an internal temperature of 165°F (74°C) is reached. Remove off the grill and set aside for a few minutes to rest.

4. Prepare the salad while the chicken is resting. Combine the mixed salad greens, cherry tomatoes, sliced red onions, crumbled feta cheese, and chopped walnuts in a large mixing basin.

5. To create the balsamic vinaigrette, mix together the balsamic vinegar, olive oil, Dijon mustard, honey, salt, and pepper in a separate small bowl.

6. Thinly slice the grilled chicken breasts.

7. Toss the salad with the balsamic vinaigrette to evenly cover the contents.

8. Divide the salad among plates and top with the grilled chicken slices.

9. Serve the grilled chicken salad for a filling and savory lunch.

Mediterranean Quinoa Bowl

Ingredients:

- 1 cup cooked quinoa
- 1 cup cherry tomatoes, halved
- 1 cucumber, diced
- 1/2 cup Kalamata olives, pitted and sliced
- 1/4 cup red onion, finely chopped
- 1/4 cup crumbled feta cheese
- 2 tablespoons chopped fresh parsley
- Juice of 1 lemon
- 2 tablespoons extra-virgin olive oil
- Salt and pepper to taste
- Optional: grilled chicken or chickpeas for added protein

Instructions:

1. Combine the cooked quinoa, cherry tomatoes, cucumber, Kalamata olives, red onion, feta cheese, and chopped parsley in a large mixing bowl.

2. To create the dressing, mix together the lemon juice, olive oil, salt, and pepper in a small bowl.

3. Toss the quinoa mixture with the dressing to coat all of the ingredients.

4. Season with salt and pepper to taste.

5. For added protein, add grilled chicken or chickpeas.

6. As a light and filling lunch alternative, serve the Mediterranean quinoa bowl.

Veggie Stir-Fry with Brown Rice

Ingredients:

- 1 cup cooked brown rice
- 1 tablespoon vegetable oil
- 1 onion, sliced

- 2 cloves garlic, minced
- 1 bell pepper, sliced
- 1 carrot, julienned
- 1 cup broccoli florets
- 1 cup snow peas
- 1 cup mushrooms, sliced
- 2 tablespoons low-sodium soy sauce
- 1 tablespoon oyster sauce (optional for non-vegetarians)
- 1 teaspoon sesame oil
- Optional: tofu or shrimp for added protein

Instructions:

1. In a large skillet or wok, heat the vegetable oil over medium-high heat.
2. Stir-fry the onion and garlic in the pan for 2-3 minutes, or until aromatic and slightly softened.
3. To the skillet, add the bell pepper, carrot, broccoli, snow peas, and mushrooms.

Stir-fry the veggies for 4-5 minutes, or until crisp-tender.

4. Whisk together the soy sauce, oyster sauce (if using), and sesame oil in a small bowl.

5. Place the cooked brown rice on one side of the pan and the veggies on the other. Stir the sauce into the rice to coat evenly.

6. Cook until the tofu or shrimp are cooked through, if preferred.

7. Mix the veggies and rice until fully mixed.

8. Remove from the heat and serve over brown rice as a filling and savory lunch choice.

Greek Salad Pita Pockets

Ingredients:

- 2 whole wheat pita pockets
- 1 cup mixed salad greens

- 1/2 cup cherry tomatoes, halved
- 1/4 cup sliced cucumber
- 1/4 cup sliced red onion
- 1/4 cup Kalamata olives, pitted and halved
- 1/4 cup crumbled feta cheese
- 2 tablespoons chopped fresh parsley
- Juice of 1/2 lemon
- 2 tablespoons extra-virgin olive oil
- Salt and pepper to taste
- Optional: grilled chicken or chickpeas for added protein.

Instructions:

1. To make pockets, cut the pita pockets in half.
2. Salad greens, cherry tomatoes, cucumber, red onion, Kalamata olives, feta cheese, and chopped parsley should all be combined in a bowl.

3. To create the dressing, mix together the lemon juice, olive oil, salt, and pepper in a small bowl.

4. Toss the salad with the dressing to coat all of the ingredients.

5. Season with salt and pepper to taste.

6. For added protein, add grilled chicken or chickpeas.

7. Fill each pita pocket halfway with the Greek salad.

8. As a light and filling lunch alternative, serve the Greek Salad Pita Pockets.

Caprese Pasta Salad

Ingredients:

- 8 ounces whole wheat pasta (such as penne or fusilli)
- 1 cup cherry tomatoes, halved
- 1 cup fresh mozzarella balls, halved
- 1/4 cup fresh basil leaves, torn

- 2 tablespoons extra-virgin olive oil
- 2 tablespoons balsamic vinegar
- Salt and pepper to taste

Instructions:

1. Cook the pasta according to package directions until it is al dente. To cool, drain and rinse with cold water.

2. Combine the cooked pasta, cherry tomatoes, fresh mozzarella balls, and broken basil leaves in a large mixing dish.

3. To create the dressing, mix together the olive oil, balsamic vinegar, salt, and pepper in a small bowl.

4. Toss the spaghetti mixture gently with the dressing to coat all of the ingredients.

5. Season with salt and pepper to taste.

6. enable the pasta salad to chill for at least 30 minutes to enable the flavors to blend.

7. Chill the Caprese Pasta Salad for a light and delightful lunch choice.

Tuna Salad Lettuce Wraps:

Ingredients:

- 2 cans tuna, drained
- 1/4 cup diced celery
- 1/4 cup diced red onion
- 2 tablespoons chopped fresh dill
- 2 tablespoons mayonnaise
- 1 tablespoon Dijon mustard
- Juice of 1/2 lemon
- Salt and pepper to taste
- Lettuce leaves for wrapping (such as romaine or butter lettuce)
- Optional toppings: sliced tomatoes, avocado, or cucumber

Instructions:

1. In a mixing dish, add the drained tuna, diced celery, diced red onion, chopped fresh dill, mayonnaise, Dijon mustard, lemon juice, salt, and pepper. Mix everything up well.

2. Season to taste.

3. Spoon the tuna salad onto each lettuce leaf.

4. Toppings such as sliced tomatoes, avocado, or cucumber may be added.

5. Roll the lettuce leaves into wraps, fastening them with toothpicks if required.

6. Serve the Tuna Salad Lettuce Wraps as a light and protein-packed lunch choice.

Veggie and Hummus Wrap

Ingredients:

- 4 whole wheat tortillas
- 1/2 cup hummus
- 1 cup mixed salad greens
- 1/2 cup shredded carrots
- 1/2 cup sliced bell peppers
- 1/2 cup sliced cucumbers

- 1/4 cup sliced red onion
- Salt and pepper to taste

Instructions:

1. Spread hummus generously on each whole wheat tortilla.
2. Toss the tortillas with the mixed salad greens, shredded carrots, sliced bell peppers, sliced cucumbers, and sliced red onion.
3. To taste, season with salt and pepper.
4. To make wraps, roll the tortillas firmly.
5. If desired, divide the wraps in half and attach them with toothpicks.
6. As a healthy and delectable lunch alternative, serve the Veggie and Hummus Wraps.

Chicken Caesar Salad

Ingredients:

- 2 boneless, skinless chicken breasts

- Salt and pepper to taste

- 8 cups romaine lettuce, chopped

- 1/4 cup grated Parmesan cheese

- 1/4 cup Caesar dressing

- 1/2 cup croutons (optional)

- Optional toppings: cherry tomatoes, sliced cucumbers, or sliced red onion

Instructions:

1. Season the chicken breasts on both sides with salt and pepper.

2. Preheat a grill or grill pan over medium-high heat. Cook the chicken breasts for 6-8 minutes each side, or until they reach an internal temperature of 165°F (74°C). Remove off the grill and let aside for a few minutes.

3. Thinly slice the grilled chicken.

4. In a large mixing bowl, combine the chopped romaine lettuce, grated Parmesan cheese, and Caesar dressing. Toss to coat the lettuce evenly.

5. Add the sliced grilled chicken and optional toppings like cherry tomatoes, sliced cucumbers, or sliced red onion.

6. Croutons may be sprinkled on top of the salad for extra crunch if desired.

7. Serve the Chicken Caesar Salad as a filling and traditional lunch choice.

Veggie Quinoa Bowl with Peanut Sauce

Ingredients:
- 1 cup cooked quinoa
- 1 cup steamed broccoli florets
- 1/2 cup shredded carrots
- 1/2 cup sliced bell peppers
- 1/2 cup edamame beans
- 1/4 cup chopped fresh cilantro
- Optional toppings: sliced green onions, sesame seeds, or crushed peanuts

- For the Peanut Sauce:

- 1/4 cup natural peanut butter

- 2 tablespoons soy sauce

- 2 tablespoons rice vinegar

- 1 tablespoon honey or maple syrup

- 1 teaspoon sesame oil

- 1/4 teaspoon grated ginger

- Water (as needed to adjust consistency)

Instructions:

1. Combine the cooked quinoa, steamed broccoli florets, shredded carrots, sliced bell peppers, edamame beans, and fresh cilantro in a mixing dish.

2. To prepare the peanut sauce, mix together the peanut butter, soy sauce, rice vinegar, honey or maple syrup, sesame oil, and chopped ginger in a separate small bowl. As required, add water gradually to adjust the sauce's consistency.

3. Distribute the peanut sauce over the quinoa-vegetable combination. Toss to evenly coat all of the ingredients.

4. Season with salt and pepper to taste.

5. Serve the vegetarian quinoa dish in individual bowls.

6. If desired, garnish with chopped green onions, sesame seeds, or crushed peanuts.

7. As a tasty and protein-rich lunch option, serve the Veggie Quinoa Bowl with Peanut Sauce.

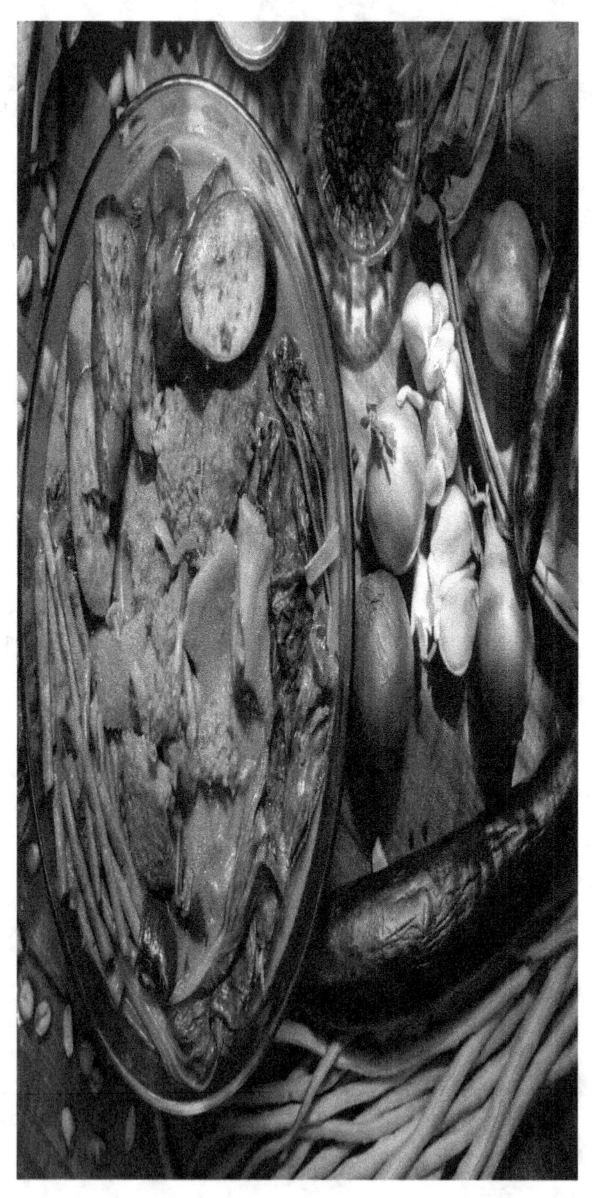

CHAPTER 3

DINNER RECIPES

Baked Salmon with Roasted Vegetables

Ingredients:

- 4 salmon fillets
- 1 pound of mixed vegetables (such as broccoli, cauliflower, carrots, and bell peppers)
- 2 tablespoons olive oil
- 2 cloves of garlic, minced
- 1 teaspoon dried thyme
- 1 teaspoon dried rosemary
- Salt and pepper to taste
- Fresh lemon wedges for serving

Instructions:

1. Preheat the oven to 425 degrees Fahrenheit (220 degrees Celsius).

2. Line a baking sheet with parchment paper and place the salmon fillets on it.

3. Combine the olive oil, minced garlic, dried thyme, dried rosemary, salt, and pepper in a small bowl.

4. Drizzle half of the oil mixture evenly over the salmon fillets.

5. Toss the mixed veggies with the remaining oil mixture in a separate dish until completely coated.

6. On a separate baking sheet, arrange the veggies in a single layer.

7. Preheat the oven to 400°F and add the fish and veggies.

8. Bake for 15-20 minutes, or until the salmon is cooked through and easily flaked with a fork, and the veggies are soft and gently browned.

9. Remove from the oven and set aside for a few minutes to cool.

10. Serve the baked salmon on a dish with roasted veggies and garnish with fresh lemon wedges for extra flavor.

11. As a healthful and filling supper alternative, serve your wonderful Baked Salmon with Roasted Vegetables.

Grilled Chicken Breast with Quinoa and Steamed Asparagus

Ingredients:

- 4 boneless, skinless chicken breasts
- 1 cup quinoa
- 2 cups water or chicken broth
- 1 bunch of asparagus, trimmed
- 2 tablespoons olive oil
- 2 cloves of garlic, minced
- 1 teaspoon dried oregano
- Salt and pepper to taste

- Lemon wedges for serving

Instructions:

1. Preheat the grill to medium-high temperature.

2. Salt, pepper, and dried oregano season the chicken breasts.

3. Bring the water or chicken broth to a boil in a saucepan. Reduce the heat to low, cover, and simmer for 15-20 minutes, or until the quinoa is tender and the liquid has been absorbed. Set aside after fluffing with a fork.

4. Steam the asparagus in a steamer basket over boiling water for 3-4 minutes, or until crisp-tender. Set aside after removing from the heat.

5. Meanwhile, in a small pan over medium heat, heat the olive oil. Sauté the minced garlic for approximately 1 minute, or until fragrant. Take the pan off the heat.

6. Cook the seasoned chicken breasts for 6-8 minutes each side on a hot grill until they reach an internal temperature of 165°F (74°C) and are no longer pink in the middle.

7. Brush the steamed asparagus with the garlic-infused olive oil and season with salt and pepper while the chicken is cooking.

8. Remove the chicken from the grill and set aside for a few minutes before slicing.

9. Serve the grilled chicken breast with some cooked quinoa and seasoned steamed asparagus.

10. Enjoy your wonderful Grilled Chicken Breast with Quinoa and Steamed Asparagus with fresh lemon juice.

Turkey Chili

Ingredients:

- 1 pound ground turkey
- 1 tablespoon olive oil
- 1 onion, chopped
- 3 cloves garlic, minced
- 1 bell pepper, chopped
- 1 can (15 ounces) kidney beans, drained and rinsed
- 1 can (15 ounces) black beans, drained and rinsed
- 1 can (15 ounces) diced tomatoes
- 1 can (6 ounces) tomato paste
- 1 cup low-sodium chicken broth
- 2 tablespoons chili powder
- 1 teaspoon ground cumin
- 1 teaspoon dried oregano
- 1/2 teaspoon paprika
- Salt and pepper to taste

- Optional toppings: shredded cheese, chopped green onions, sour cream, cilantro

Instructions:

1. In a large saucepan or Dutch oven, heat the olive oil over medium heat.

2. Cook, breaking up the ground turkey with a spoon, until it is browned and cooked through.

3. To the saucepan, add the chopped onion, minced garlic, and bell pepper. Cook for 5 minutes, or until the veggies have softened.

4. To the saucepan, include the kidney beans, black beans, chopped tomatoes (with juices), tomato paste, chicken stock, chili powder, cumin, oregano, paprika, salt, and pepper. To blend, stir everything together well.

5. Bring the chili to a boil and cook for 20-30 minutes, stirring periodically.

6. Adjust the seasoning with salt and pepper to taste.

7. Serve the turkey chili hot, topped with your preferred toppings such as shredded cheese, chopped green onions, sour cream, and cilantro.

8. Enjoy your tasty and warming Turkey Chili!

Cauliflower Fried Rice with Shrimp

Ingredients:

- 1 medium cauliflower head
- 1 pound shrimp, peeled and deveined
- 2 tablespoons vegetable oil
- 2 cloves garlic, minced
- 1 small onion, finely chopped
- 1 carrot, diced
- 1 cup frozen peas
- 2 tablespoons low-sodium soy sauce
- 1 tablespoon sesame oil

- 2 eggs, beaten

- Salt and pepper to taste

- Optional toppings: chopped green onions, sesame seeds

Instructions:

1. Remove the stalks from the cauliflower and cut it into florets. In a food processor, pulse the florets until they resemble rice grains.

2. In a large skillet or wok, heat 1 tablespoon vegetable oil over medium-high heat.

3. Cook the shrimp for 2-3 minutes on each side, or until they become pink and opaque. Take the shrimp out of the pan and put aside.

4. Heat another tablespoon of vegetable oil in the same skillet.

5. To the skillet, add the minced garlic, chopped onion, and diced carrot. Sauté

for 3-4 minutes, or until the veggies soften.

6. In the skillet, combine the cauliflower rice and frozen peas. Stir-fry for 5 minutes, or until the cauliflower is tender-crisp and the peas are warm.

7. Whisk together the low-sodium soy sauce and sesame oil in a small bowl. Pour the sauce over the cauliflower rice mixture and toss to coat evenly.

8. Make an empty space in the pan by pushing the cauliflower rice mixture to one side.

9. Scramble the beaten eggs in the empty area until they are thoroughly cooked.

10. Return the cooked shrimp to the pan and toss everything together.

11. Season to taste with salt and pepper.

12. Remove from heat and, if preferred, sprinkle with chopped green onions and sesame seeds.

13. As a tasty and healthful alternative to classic fried rice, serve the Cauliflower Fried Rice with Shrimp hot.

Baked Cod with Lemon and Herbs

Ingredients:

- 4 cod fillets
- 2 tablespoons olive oil
- 2 tablespoons fresh lemon juice
- 1 teaspoon dried thyme
- 1 teaspoon dried parsley
- 1 teaspoon dried dill
- 1/2 teaspoon garlic powder
- Salt and pepper to taste
- Fresh lemon slices for garnish

Instructions:

1. Preheat oven to 400°F (200°C).
2. Put the fish fillets in a baking dish lined with parchment paper.

3. In a small bowl, mix together the olive oil, lemon juice, dried thyme, dried parsley, dried dill, garlic powder, salt, and pepper.

4. Drizzle the herb and lemon mixture over the cod fillets, ensuring sure they're uniformly covered.

5. Top each fish fillet with fresh lemon slices for extra flavor.

6. Bake the cod in a preheated oven for 12-15 minutes, or until it is opaque and flakes readily with a fork.

7. Remove from the oven and rest for a few minutes before serving.

8. Serve the Baked Cod with Lemon and Herbs hot, topped with more fresh lemon slices.

9. For a full dinner, serve it with steamed veggies and a side of brown rice or quinoa.

Beef Stir-Fry with Brown Rice

Ingredients:

- 1 pound beef sirloin, thinly sliced
- 2 tablespoons soy sauce
- 2 tablespoons oyster sauce
- 1 tablespoon cornstarch
- 1 tablespoon vegetable oil
- 3 cloves garlic, minced
- 1-inch piece of ginger, grated
- 1 onion, sliced
- 1 bell pepper, sliced
- 1 cup sliced mushrooms
- 2 cups broccoli florets
- 2 cups cooked brown rice
- Salt and pepper to taste
- Optional toppings: sliced green onions, sesame seeds

Instructions:

1. In a bowl, combine the thinly sliced beef, soy sauce, oyster sauce, and cornstarch.

Stir well to coat the beef evenly. Let it marinate for about 15-20 minutes.

2. Heat the vegetable oil in a large skillet or wok over high heat.

3. Add the minced garlic and grated ginger to the skillet. Sauté for about 1 minute until fragrant.

4. Add the marinated beef to the skillet and stir-fry for about 2-3 minutes until the beef is browned and cooked through. Remove the beef from the skillet and set aside.

5. In the same skillet, add the sliced onion, bell pepper, and mushrooms. Stir-fry for about 3-4 minutes until the vegetables start to soften.

6. Add the broccoli florets to the skillet and continue stir-frying for another 2-3 minutes until the broccoli is tender-crisp.

7. Return the cooked beef to the skillet and stir everything together to combine.

8. Season with salt and pepper to taste.

9. Serve the beef stir-fry over a bed of cooked brown rice.

10. Garnish with sliced green onions and sesame seeds, if desired.

11. Enjoy your flavorful and nutritious Beef Stir-Fry with Brown Rice!

Stuffed Bell Peppers with Lean Ground Beef and Quinoa

Ingredients:

- 4 bell peppers (any color)
- 1 pound lean ground beef
- 1 cup cooked quinoa
- 1 small onion, finely chopped
- 2 cloves garlic, minced
- 1 can (14 ounces) diced tomatoes, drained
- 1 cup shredded mozzarella cheese

- 2 tablespoons tomato paste

- 1 teaspoon dried oregano

- 1 teaspoon dried basil

- Salt and pepper to taste

- Fresh parsley for garnish

Instructions:

1. Preheat the oven to 375°F (190°C).

2. Cut the tops off the bell peppers and remove the seeds and membranes. Set aside.

3. In a large skillet, cook the lean ground beef over medium heat until browned and cooked through. Drain any excess fat.

4. Add the chopped onion and minced garlic to the skillet with the cooked ground beef. Sauté for about 3-4 minutes until the onion is translucent.

5. Stir in the cooked quinoa, diced tomatoes, tomato paste, dried oregano, dried basil, salt, and pepper. Cook for

another 2-3 minutes until everything is well combined and heated through.

6. Spoon the beef and quinoa mixture into the hollowed-out bell peppers, filling them evenly.

7. Place the stuffed bell peppers in a baking dish and cover with foil.

8. Bake in the preheated oven for about 25-30 minutes until the bell peppers are tender.

9. Remove the foil and sprinkle the shredded mozzarella cheese over the top of each stuffed bell pepper.

10. Return the baking dish to the oven and bake for an additional 5 minutes or until the cheese is melted and bubbly.

11. Remove from the oven and let the stuffed bell peppers cool for a few minutes.

12. Garnish with fresh parsley and serve the Stuffed Bell Peppers with Lean Ground

Beef and Quinoa as a satisfying and nutritious meal.

Veggie and Chickpea Curry:

Ingredients:

- 1 tablespoon vegetable oil
- 1 onion, chopped
- 3 cloves garlic, minced
- 1-inch piece of ginger, grated
- 1 tablespoon curry powder
- 1 teaspoon ground cumin
- 1 teaspoon ground coriander
- 1/2 teaspoon turmeric
- 1/4 teaspoon cayenne pepper (optional, for added heat)
- 1 can (14 ounces) diced tomatoes
- 1 can (14 ounces) coconut milk
- 1 can (14 ounces) chickpeas, drained and rinsed

- 2 cups mixed vegetables (such as bell peppers, carrots, peas, and cauliflower), chopped
- Salt and pepper to taste
- Fresh cilantro for garnish
- Cooked rice or naan bread for serving

Instructions:

1. In a large skillet or saucepan, heat the vegetable oil over medium heat.
2. Sauté the chopped onion in the pan for approximately 5 minutes, or until it turns translucent.
3. To the skillet, add the minced garlic and grated ginger. Cook for a another 1-2 minutes, or until fragrant.
4. Combine the curry powder, ground cumin, ground coriander, turmeric, and cayenne pepper (if using) in a small bowl. To make a spice combination, stir everything together.

5. Stir the spice mixture into the skillet to coat the onions, garlic, and ginger.

6. Add the chopped tomatoes (with liquids) and coconut milk. Stir everything together.

7. To the pan, add the drained and rinsed chickpeas and chopped mixed veggies. Stir them in the curry sauce to coat.

8. Reduce the heat to low, cover the pan, and cook for 15-20 minutes, or until the veggies are soft.

9. Season to taste with salt and pepper.

10. Serve the Veggie and Chickpea Curry hot with rice or naan bread.

11. Garnish with fresh cilantro leaves for extra taste and freshness.

12. Enjoy your tasty and warming Veggie and Chickpea Curry!

Lentil Soup with Spinach and Tomatoes:

Ingredients:

- 1 tablespoon olive oil
- 1 onion, chopped
- 3 cloves garlic, minced
- 1 carrot, diced
- 1 celery stalk, diced
- 1 cup dried lentils (green or brown), rinsed and drained
- 1 can (14 ounces) diced tomatoes
- 4 cups vegetable broth
- 2 cups fresh spinach leaves, chopped
- 1 teaspoon ground cumin
- 1 teaspoon ground paprika
- 1/2 teaspoon dried thyme
- Salt and pepper to taste
- Fresh lemon wedges for serving

Instructions:

1. In a large saucepan over medium heat, heat the olive oil.

2. To the saucepan, add the chopped onion, minced garlic, diced carrot, and diced celery. Cook for 5 minutes, or until the veggies soften.

3. To the saucepan, include the washed lentils, chopped tomatoes (with juices), vegetable broth, ground cumin, ground paprika, dried thyme, salt, and pepper. Stir everything together well.

4. Bring the soup to a boil, then lower to a low heat and cover. Allow the soup to boil for 25-30 minutes, or until the lentils are cooked.

5. Stir the chopped spinach leaves into the broth until they have wilted.

6. Adjust the seasoning with salt and pepper to taste.

7. Remove from the heat and set aside to cool slightly before serving.

8. Pour the Lentil Soup with Spinach and Tomatoes into individual bowls.

9. Serve with fresh lemon wedges on the side for squeezing over the soup for added freshness and tanginess.

10. Enjoy your hearty and filling Lentil Soup with Spinach and Tomatoes!

Grilled Steak with Roasted Cauliflower Mash

Ingredients:

- 2 steaks (such as ribeye, sirloin, or filet mignon)
- Salt and pepper to taste
- 1 head cauliflower, cut into florets
- 2 tablespoons olive oil
- 2 cloves garlic, minced
- 1/4 cup grated Parmesan cheese
- 1/4 cup unsweetened almond milk (or regular milk)
- 2 tablespoons butter

- Fresh parsley for garnish

Instructions:

1. Preheat the grill to medium-high heat.

2. Season the steaks generously with salt and pepper on both sides.

3. Place the seasoned steaks on the grill and cook to your desired doneness, typically about 4-6 minutes per side for medium-rare. Adjust the cooking time based on your preference and the thickness of the steaks.

4. Remove the steaks from the grill and let them rest for a few minutes before slicing.

5. Meanwhile, preheat the oven to 400°F (200°C).

6. In a large bowl, toss the cauliflower florets with olive oil, minced garlic, salt, and pepper.

7. Spread the cauliflower florets in a single layer on a baking sheet lined with parchment paper.

8. Roast the cauliflower in the preheated oven for about 25-30 minutes until they are tender and lightly browned.

9. Transfer the roasted cauliflower to a food processor or blender. Add the grated Parmesan cheese, almond milk, and butter.

10. Blend the ingredients until smooth and creamy, adjusting the consistency with more almond milk if needed.

11. Season the cauliflower mash with additional salt and pepper to taste.

12. Slice the grilled steaks and serve them alongside the roasted cauliflower mash.

13. Garnish with fresh parsley for added freshness and presentation.

14. Enjoy your delicious and satisfying Grilled Steak with Roasted Cauliflower Mash!

Ingredients:

- 4 bone-in, skin-on chicken thighs
- 2 tablespoons olive oil
- 1 tablespoon paprika
- 1 teaspoon garlic powder
- 1 teaspoon dried thyme
- Salt and pepper to taste
- 2 large sweet potatoes, peeled and cut into cubes
- 1 tablespoon melted butter
- 1 tablespoon honey
- Fresh parsley for garnish

Instructions:

1. Preheating the oven to 400°F (200°C) is recommended.

2. To create the marinade, whisk together the olive oil, paprika, garlic powder,

dried thyme, salt, and pepper in a small bowl.

3. Place the chicken thighs in a baking dish and brush both sides with the marinade.

4. In the baking dish, arrange the sweet potato cubes around the chicken thighs.

5. Drizzle the sweet potatoes with the melted butter and honey, then season with salt & pepper to taste.

6. Bake for 35-40 minutes, or until the chicken thighs are cooked through and the sweet potatoes are soft in a preheated oven.

7. Allow the baking dish to cool for a few minutes after taking it out of the oven.

8. To enhance freshness and appearance, garnish with fresh parsley.

9. Serve the Baked Chicken Thighs with the Roasted Sweet Potatoes for a filling and nutritious supper.

CHAPTER 4

Snacks and appetizers

Veggie Sticks with Hummus:

Ingredients:

- Assorted raw vegetables such as carrot sticks, cucumber slices, bell pepper strips, and celery sticks.
- Store-bought or homemade hummus for dipping.

Instructions:

1. Wash and prepare the vegetables by cutting them into sticks or slices.
2. Arrange the vegetable sticks on a serving platter or plate.
3. Place a bowl of hummus in the center of the platter.

4. Serve the veggie sticks alongside the hummus, allowing guests to dip the vegetables into the hummus.

5. Enjoy the crunchy and refreshing Veggie Sticks with Hummus as a healthy and flavorful snack or appetizer.

Greek Yogurt with Berries:

Ingredients:

- 1 cup plain Greek yogurt (low-fat or non-fat)
- 1/2 cup fresh berries (such as blueberries, raspberries, or strawberries)
- 1/2 teaspoon honey or a natural sweetener (optional)
- A sprinkle of cinnamon (optional)

Instructions:

1. Scoop the Greek yogurt into a bowl or serving plate.

2. Rinse and pat dry the fresh berries with cool water.

3. Top the Greek yogurt with the fresh berries.

4. If preferred, drizzle a spoonful of honey or a natural sweetener over the berries.

5. To enhance flavor, sprinkle a touch of cinnamon on top.

6. Gently combine the ingredients, making sure the berries are uniformly distributed.

7. Serve the Greek Yogurt with Berries as a tasty and nutritious snack or breakfast alternative.

8. Enjoy the creamy yogurt and the luscious berries' blast of flavor.

Baked Parmesan Zucchini Chips:

Ingredients:

- 2 medium zucchini
- 1/4 cup grated Parmesan cheese

- 1/4 teaspoon garlic powder

- 1/4 teaspoon paprika

- Salt and pepper to taste

- Cooking spray or olive oil

Instructions:

1. Preheat the oven to 425 degrees Fahrenheit (220 degrees Celsius) and line a baking sheet with parchment paper.

2. Wash the zucchini and cut it into thin slices about a quarter-inch thick. To eliminate any extra moisture, pat them dry with a paper towel.

3. Combine the grated Parmesan cheese, garlic powder, paprika, salt, and pepper in a small bowl. Combine thoroughly.

4. To avoid sticking, lightly coat or brush the prepared baking sheet with cooking spray.

5. Place the zucchini slices in a single layer on the baking sheet, ensuring sure they do not overlap.

6. Sprinkle the Parmesan cheese mixture evenly over the zucchini slices, being sure to cover each one.

7. Bake for 15-20 minutes, or until the zucchini chips are golden and crispy, in a preheated oven.

8. Remove from the oven and set aside to cool before serving.

9. Baked Parmesan Zucchini Chips are a tasty and healthful snack.

Avocado Deviled Eggs:

Ingredients:

- 6 hard-boiled eggs
- 1 ripe avocado
- 1 tablespoon Greek yogurt or mayonnaise

- 1 teaspoon Dijon mustard

- 1 teaspoon lime juice

- Salt and pepper to taste

- Optional garnish: Paprika or chopped chives

Instructions:

1. Peel the hard-boiled eggs carefully and cut them in half lengthwise. Separate the yolks and set them aside in a separate dish.

2. Remove the pit from the avocado and spoon the flesh into the dish with the egg yolks.

3. Combine the egg yolks and avocado until fully mixed and creamy.

4. Mix in the Greek yogurt or mayonnaise, Dijon mustard, lime juice, salt, and pepper. To blend, stir everything together well.

5. If necessary, taste the filling and adjust the spice.

6. Fill the egg white halves with the avocado deviled egg filling, dividing it equally.

7. For extra taste and appearance, sprinkle paprika or chopped chives on top of each deviled egg.

8. enable the Avocado Deviled Eggs to chill for at least 30 minutes before serving to enable the flavors to mingle.

9. Serve these creamy and savory Avocado Deviled Eggs chilled as an appetizer or snack.

Cucumber and Tuna Bites:

Ingredients:

- 1 English cucumber
- 1 can of tuna in water, drained
- 2 tablespoons Greek yogurt or mayonnaise
- 1 teaspoon lemon juice

- 1 tablespoon chopped fresh dill or parsley (optional)
- Salt and pepper to taste
- Optional garnish: Slices of cherry tomato or black olives

Instructions:

1. Wash the English cucumber and cut it into 1/2-inch thick rounds.
2. Combine the drained tuna, Greek yogurt or mayonnaise, lemon juice, fresh dill or parsley (if using), salt, and pepper in a mixing dish. To mix, integrate everything thoroughly.
3. Adjust the seasoning to taste with the tuna mixture.
4. Using a spoon, make a tiny indentation in the middle of a cucumber round. This will provide a hollow hole for the tuna filling.
5. Fill each cucumber round with a tablespoon of the tuna mixture, carefully

pushing it down to form a bite-sized piece.

6. Optional: Add a slice of cherry tomato or a tiny sliver of black olive to each cucumber and tuna mouthful.

7. Place the Cucumber and Tuna Bites on a serving dish and place in the refrigerator for at least 15 minutes to enable the flavors to mingle.

8. Serve chilled as a nutritious and refreshing appetizer or snack.

Roasted Chickpeas:

Ingredients:

- 1 can (15 ounces) chickpeas (garbanzo beans)
- 1 tablespoon olive oil
- 1/2 teaspoon ground cumin
- 1/2 teaspoon paprika
- 1/2 teaspoon garlic powder

- 1/4 teaspoon salt

- Optional: Pinch of cayenne pepper or other desired spices

Instructions:

1. Preheat the oven to 400 degrees Fahrenheit (200 degrees Celsius) and line a baking sheet with parchment paper.

2. After draining and rinsing the chickpeas, blot them dry with a paper towel to eliminate any extra moisture.

3. Toss the chickpeas in a bowl with the olive oil, cumin, paprika, garlic powder, salt, and any other spices you like. Check that the chickpeas are uniformly coated.

4. On the prepared baking sheet, spread the seasoned chickpeas in a single layer.

5. Cook the chickpeas in a preheated oven for 25-30 minutes, or until crispy and golden brown. To achieve consistent

browning, stir the chickpeas once or twice while cooking.

6. Remove the baking sheet from the oven and set aside for a few minutes to cool.

7. Roasted Chickpeas are a crispy, protein-rich snack.

8. For a few days, store any leftovers in an airtight jar at room temperature.

Mini Caprese Skewers:

Ingredients:

- Cherry tomatoes
- Fresh mozzarella balls (bocconcini)
- Fresh basil leaves
- Balsamic glaze or balsamic reduction
- Toothpicks or small skewers

Instructions:

1. Rinse and pat dry the cherry tomatoes with a paper towel.

2. If necessary, drain the fresh mozzarella balls.

3. Thread a cherry tomato onto a toothpick or tiny skewer.

4. Then add a fresh basil leaf, folded or split in half, and a mozzarella ball.

5. Repeat until you have created the necessary number of small caprese skewers.

6. Place the small caprese skewers on a serving plate and serve.

7. Drizzle balsamic glaze or balsamic reduction over the skewers.

8. Optional: For presentation, garnish the tray with additional fresh basil leaves.

9. Mini Caprese Skewers are a tasty and colorful appetizer or snack.

Almond Butter and Apple Slices:

Ingredients:

- 1 apple (any variety you prefer)
- 2 tablespoons almond butter
- Optional toppings: Cinnamon, honey, or chopped nuts

Instructions:

1. Wash and dry the apple with a paper towel.

2. Cut the apple into small pieces after core it.

3. On each apple slice, spread a thin coating of almond butter.

4. Optional: For extra taste and texture, sprinkle a bit of cinnamon, a drizzle of honey, or some chopped nuts on top of the almond butter.

5. Arrange the Apple Slices with Almond Butter on a dish or serving tray.

6. Serve immediately as a nutritious and filling snack.

Mini Vegetable Frittatas

Ingredients:

- 6 large eggs
- 1/4 cup milk (or dairy-free milk alternative)
- 1/2 cup diced vegetables (such as bell peppers, spinach, onions, mushrooms, or any vegetables of your choice)
- 1/4 cup shredded cheese (such as cheddar, mozzarella, or feta)
- Salt and pepper to taste
- Cooking spray or olive oil

Instructions:

1. Preheat your oven to 375°F (190°C) and lightly grease a muffin tin with cooking spray or olive oil.

2. In a bowl, whisk together the eggs and milk until well beaten.

3. Add the diced vegetables, shredded cheese, salt, and pepper to the egg mixture. Stir to combine.

4. Pour the egg and vegetable mixture evenly into each muffin cup, filling them about 3/4 full.

5. Optional: You can sprinkle some extra cheese on top of each frittata for added flavor.

6. Bake in the preheated oven for about 20-25 minutes or until the frittatas are set and slightly golden on top.

7. Remove the muffin tin from the oven and let the frittatas cool for a few minutes.

8. Carefully remove the mini vegetable frittatas from the muffin tin using a spoon or knife.

9. Serve the Mini Vegetable Frittatas warm or at room temperature as a delicious and nutritious snack or light meal.

Guacamole with Baked Tortilla Chips:

Ingredients for Guacamole:

- 2 ripe avocados
- 1 small onion, finely chopped
- 1 tomato, diced
- 1 jalapeño pepper, seeded and finely chopped (optional)
- 2 tablespoons fresh lime juice
- 2 tablespoons chopped fresh cilantro
- Salt and pepper to taste

Ingredients for Baked Tortilla Chips:

- 6 whole wheat tortillas
- Olive oil spray or cooking spray
- Salt to taste

Instructions for Guacamole:

1. Remove the pits from the avocados and spoon the flesh into a basin.

2. With a fork, mash the avocados until smooth, or leave them slightly chunky if preferred.

3. To the mashed avocados, add the chopped onion, diced tomato, jalapeo pepper (if using), lime juice, chopped cilantro, salt, and pepper.

4. Stir in all of the ingredients until fully blended.

5. Adjust the spice to taste with the guacamole.

6. Refrigerate the guacamole in a serving dish, covered with plastic wrap, until ready to serve.

Instructions Baked Tortilla Chips:

1. Preheat the oven to 350 degrees Fahrenheit (175 degrees Celsius).

2. Cut each tortilla into wedges or other shapes as desired.

3. Arrange the tortilla wedges on a baking sheet in a single layer.

4. Spray the tortilla wedges lightly with olive oil spray or cooking spray.

5. Season the tortilla wedges with salt.

6. Bake for 10-12 minutes, or until the tortilla chips are crispy and golden brown, in a preheated oven.

7. Allow the cooked tortilla chips to cool fully before serving.

Greek Salad Skewers:

Ingredients:

- Cherry tomatoes
- Cucumber, cut into cubes
- Kalamata olives, pitted
- Feta cheese, cut into cubes

- Red onion, cut into small wedges

- Fresh basil leaves

- Wooden skewers

Instructions:

1. Rinse the cherry tomatoes, cucumber, and basil leaves before assembling the dish. Using a paper towel, pat them dry.

2. Thread the ingredients in whichever order you choose onto the wooden skewers. Begin with a cherry tomato, then add a cucumber cube, a folded basil leaf, a feta cheese cube, a Kalamata olive, and a slice of red onion. Repeat the procedure until the skewer is finished.

3. Continue making the Greek Salad Skewers until you have the appropriate number.

4. Arrange the skewers on a dish to serve.

5. Drizzle some olive oil and sprinkle some dried oregano over the skewers for more flavor.

6. Serve the Greek Salad Skewers as a light and refreshing appetizer or party snack.

Smoked Salmon Roll-ups:

Ingredients:

- Sliced smoked salmon
- Cream cheese (plain or flavored, such as dill or chive)
- Cucumber, cut into thin strips
- Fresh dill, chopped
- Lemon zest (optional)
- Toothpicks

Instructions:

1. Place a smoked salmon slice on a clean surface.

2. Spread smoked salmon slices with a thin layer of cream cheese.

3. On one end of the salmon slice, arrange a few cucumber slices horizontally.

4. Sprinkle the cream cheese and cucumber with chopped fresh dill and a dash of lemon zest (if using).

5. Roll up the smoked salmon firmly, beginning with the cucumber.

6. Insert a toothpick into the end of the roll to secure it.

7. Rep with the rest of the smoked salmon pieces and ingredients.

8. Serve the Smoked Salmon Roll-ups on a tray.

9. Optional: For presentation, garnish the plate with more fresh dill.

10. As an elegant and savory appetizer or light snack, serve the Smoked Salmon Roll-ups.

CHAPTER 5

SMOOTHIES

Berry Blast Smoothie:

- 1 cup mixed berries (strawberries, blueberries, raspberries)
- 1/2 cup unsweetened almond milk
- 1/4 cup Greek yogurt (plain or unsweetened)
- 1 tablespoon ground flaxseed
- 1 teaspoon honey (optional for added sweetness)
- Ice cubes (optional)

Green Power Smoothie:

- 1 cup spinach
- 1/2 medium cucumber, peeled and sliced
- 1/2 ripe avocado
- 1/2 medium banana

- 1/2 cup unsweetened coconut water

- Juice of 1/2 lemon

- Ice cubes (optional)

Tropical Paradise Smoothie:

- 1/2 cup frozen mango chunks

- 1/2 cup frozen pineapple chunks

- 1/2 medium banana

- 1/2 cup unsweetened coconut milk

- 1/4 cup Greek yogurt (plain or unsweetened)

- 1 tablespoon chia seeds

- Ice cubes (optional)

Creamy Almond Butter Smoothie:

- 1 cup unsweetened almond milk

- 2 tablespoons almond butter

- 1/2 medium banana

- 1/4 teaspoon cinnamon

- 1/4 teaspoon vanilla extract

- Ice cubes (optional)

Cinnamon Apple Pie Smoothie:

- 1 medium apple, cored and chopped
- 1/2 cup unsweetened almond milk
- 1/4 cup Greek yogurt (plain or unsweetened)
- 1 tablespoon almond butter
- 1/2 teaspoon cinnamon
- Ice cubes (optional)

Creamy Blueberry Smoothie:

- 1 cup frozen blueberries
- 1/2 cup unsweetened almond milk
- 1/4 cup Greek yogurt (plain or unsweetened)
- 1 tablespoon almond butter
- 1 tablespoon ground flaxseed
- Ice cubes (optional)

Veggie Power Smoothie:

- 1/2 cup baby spinach
- 1/2 medium cucumber, peeled and sliced
- 1/2 medium carrot, peeled and chopped
- 1/2 medium banana
- 1/2 cup unsweetened almond milk
- Juice of 1/2 lemon
- Ice cubes (optional)

Chocolate Banana Smoothie:

- 1/2 medium banana
- 1 tablespoon unsweetened cocoa powder
- 1 cup unsweetened almond milk
- 1/4 cup Greek yogurt (plain or unsweetened)
- 1 tablespoon almond butter
- Ice cubes (optional)

Ginger Turmeric Smoothie:

- 1 cup unsweetened almond milk
- 1/2 teaspoon grated fresh ginger
- 1/2 teaspoon ground turmeric
- 1/2 medium banana
- 1 tablespoon chia seeds
- 1 teaspoon honey (optional for added sweetness)
- Ice cubes (optional)

Pineapple Coconut Smoothie:

- 1 cup frozen pineapple chunks
- 1/2 cup unsweetened coconut milk
- 1/4 cup Greek yogurt (plain or unsweetened)
- 1 tablespoon unsweetened shredded coconut
- 1 tablespoon ground flaxseed
- Ice cubes (optional)

Minty Green Smoothie:

- 1 cup baby spinach
- 1/2 medium cucumber, peeled and sliced
- 1/2 medium avocado
- 1/2 cup unsweetened almond milk
- 1 tablespoon fresh mint leaves
- Juice of 1/2 lime
- Ice cubes (optional)

Pomegranate Berry Smoothie:

- 1/2 cup frozen mixed berries (strawberries, blueberries, raspberries)
- 1/4 cup pomegranate juice (unsweetened)
- 1/2 cup unsweetened almond milk
- 1/4 cup Greek yogurt (plain or unsweetened)
- 1 tablespoon chia seeds
- Ice cubes (optional)

Mango Turmeric Smoothie:

- 1 cup frozen mango chunks
- 1/2 teaspoon ground turmeric
- 1/2 teaspoon grated fresh ginger
- 1 cup unsweetened almond milk
- 1/4 cup Greek yogurt (plain or unsweetened)
- 1 tablespoon ground flaxseed
- Ice cubes (optional)

Coffee Protein Smoothie:

- 1 cup brewed coffee, cooled
- 1/2 cup unsweetened almond milk
- 1/4 cup Greek yogurt (plain or unsweetened)
- 1 tablespoon almond butter
- 1 scoop protein powder (choose a low-sugar option)
- Ice cubes (optional)

Coconut Berry Smoothie:

- 1/2 cup frozen mixed berries (strawberries, blueberries, raspberries)
- 1/4 cup unsweetened coconut milk
- 1/2 cup unsweetened almond milk
- 1/4 cup Greek yogurt (plain or unsweetened)
- 1 tablespoon unsweetened shredded coconut
- 1 tablespoon ground flaxseed
- Ice cubes (optional)

Banana Walnut Smoothie:

- 1 medium banana
- 2 tablespoons walnuts
- 1 cup unsweetened almond milk
- 1/4 cup Greek yogurt (plain or unsweetened)
- 1 tablespoon almond butter

- 1 teaspoon honey (optional for added sweetness)
- Ice cubes (optional)

Citrus Spinach Smoothie:

- 1 cup baby spinach
- 1/2 medium orange, peeled and segmented
- 1/2 medium banana
- 1/2 cup unsweetened orange juice
- 1/4 cup Greek yogurt (plain or unsweetened)
- 1 tablespoon chia seeds
- Ice cubes (optional)

Apple Cinnamon Smoothie:

- 1 medium apple, cored and chopped
- 1/2 teaspoon ground cinnamon
- 1 cup unsweetened almond milk

- 1/4 cup Greek yogurt (plain or unsweetened)
- 1 tablespoon almond butter
- 1 tablespoon ground flaxseed
- Ice cubes (optional)

Green Apple and Kale Smoothie:

- 1 medium green apple, cored and chopped
- 1 cup chopped kale leaves
- 1/2 medium banana
- 1/2 cup unsweetened almond milk
- 1/4 cup Greek yogurt (plain or unsweetened)
- 1 tablespoon almond butter
- Ice cubes (optional)

NOTE: Instructions for all smoothies:

Place all the ingredients in a blender.

Blend on high until smooth and creamy.

If desired, add ice cubes and blend again for a thicker and colder smoothie.

PpPour into a glass and enjoy immediately.

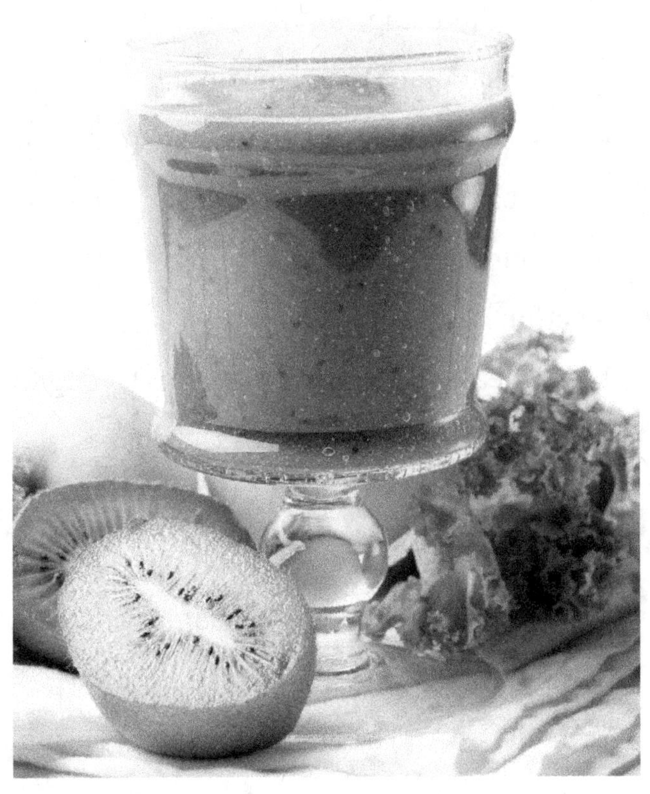

CHAPTER 6

DESSERTS

Baked Apples with Cinnamon:

Ingredients:

- 2 medium apples
- 1 teaspoon ground cinnamon
- 1 tablespoon chopped walnuts (optional)
- 1 teaspoon honey or sugar substitute (optional)

Instructions:

1. Preheat the oven to 350 degrees Fahrenheit (175 degrees Celsius).
2. Place the apples in a baking dish and core them.
3. If desired, sprinkle cinnamon over the apples and top with chopped walnuts.
4. If desired, drizzle with honey or sprinkle with a sugar alternative.

5. Bake the apples for 25-30 minutes, or until soft.

6. Serve warm with a dollop of Greek yogurt if desired.

Dark Chocolate-Dipped Strawberries:

Ingredients:

- Fresh strawberries
- Dark chocolate (at least 70% cocoa)
- Instructions:
- Wash and dry the strawberries.
- Melt the dark chocolate in a microwave-safe bowl, stirring every 30 seconds until smooth.
- Dip each strawberry into the melted chocolate, coating it about halfway.
- Place the dipped strawberries on a parchment-lined baking sheet.

- Let the chocolate set at room temperature or refrigerate for a few minutes until firm.
- Enjoy the delicious combination of dark chocolate and strawberries.
-
- Greek Yogurt Parfait:
- Ingredients:
- 1 cup Greek yogurt (plain or unsweetened)
- Fresh berries (strawberries, blueberries, raspberries)
- 1 tablespoon chopped nuts (e.g., almonds, walnuts)
- 1 teaspoon honey or sugar substitute (optional)

Instructions:

1. Layer Greek yogurt, fresh berries, and chopped almonds in a glass or dish.
2. Repeat the layering until all of the ingredients have been utilized.

3. If desired, drizzle with honey or sprinkle with a sugar alternative.

4. As a refreshing treat, serve the creamy and fruity parfait.

Chia Seed Pudding:

Ingredients:

- 1/4 cup chia seeds
- 1 cup unsweetened almond milk
- 1 teaspoon vanilla extract
- 1 tablespoon honey or sugar substitute (optional)
- Fresh berries or sliced fruits for topping
- Instructions:
- Combine chia seeds, almond milk, vanilla essence, and honey or sugar alternative in a mixing dish.
- Stir carefully to disperse the chia seeds evenly.

- Allow the mixture to settle for 5 minutes before stirring again to avoid clumping.
- Cover and place in the refrigerator for at least 2 hours or overnight.
- Serve chilled chia seed pudding with fresh berries or sliced fruits on top.
- Berry Yogurt Popsicles:
- Ingredients:
- 1 cup mixed berries (strawberries, blueberries, raspberries)
- 1 cup Greek yogurt (plain or unsweetened)
- 1 tablespoon honey or sugar substitute (optional)

Instructions:

1. Blend the mixed berries in a blender until smooth.
2. In a bowl, mix the blended berries with Greek yogurt and honey or sugar substitute.

3. Pour the mixture into popsicle molds and insert popsicle sticks.

4. Freeze for at least 4 hours or until firm.

5. Enjoy these refreshing and fruity popsicles on a hot day.

Peanut Butter Banana Ice Cream:

Ingredients:

- 2 ripe bananas, peeled and sliced
- 2 tablespoons natural peanut butter

Instructions:

1. Place the sliced bananas in a ziplock bag and freeze for at least 2 hours.

2. Once frozen, transfer the bananas to a blender or food processor.

3. Add the peanut butter and blend until smooth and creamy.

4. Serve immediately as soft-serve ice cream or transfer to a container and freeze for a firmer texture.

5. Indulge in this creamy and guilt-free ice cream alternative.

Baked Pears with Cinnamon and Almonds:

Ingredients:

- 2 ripe pears, halved and cored
- 1 tablespoon melted coconut oil or butter
- 1 teaspoon ground cinnamon
- 2 tablespoons chopped almonds
- 1 teaspoon honey or sugar substitute (optional)

Instructions:

1. Preheat the oven to 350 degrees Fahrenheit (175 degrees Celsius).
2. Place the pear halves cut side up on a baking sheet.

3. Brush the pears with the melted coconut oil or butter.

4. Sprinkle cinnamon and almonds on top of each pear half.

5. If desired, drizzle with honey or sprinkle with a sugar alternative.

6. Bake the pears for 20-25 minutes, or until they are soft.

7. As a delectable dessert, serve these warm and soothing baked pears.

Coconut Chia Pudding with Berries:

Ingredients:

- 1/4 cup chia seeds
- 1 cup unsweetened coconut milk
- 1 tablespoon unsweetened shredded coconut
- 1 teaspoon vanilla extract
- Fresh berries for topping

Instructions:

1. Combine the chia seeds, coconut milk,
    shredded coconut, and vanilla essence in
    a mixing dish.
2. Stir carefully to disperse the chia seeds
    evenly.
3. Allow the mixture to settle for 5 minutes
    before stirring again to avoid clumping.
4. Cover and place in the refrigerator for at
    least 2 hours or overnight.
5. Serve the cooled chia pudding with fresh
    berries on top.

Cinnamon Baked Apples with Yogurt:

Ingredients:

- 2 medium apples
- 1 teaspoon ground cinnamon
- 2 tablespoons chopped nuts (e.g., almonds, walnuts)

- 1 cup Greek yogurt (plain or unsweetened)

Instructions:

1. Preheat the oven to 350 degrees Fahrenheit (175 degrees Celsius).
2. Place the apples in a baking dish and core them.
3. Sprinkle cinnamon and chopped nuts over the apples.
4. Bake the apples for 25-30 minutes, or until soft.
5. Warm with a dollop of Greek yogurt on top.

Dark Chocolate Bark with Almonds:

Ingredients:

- 3 ounces dark chocolate (at least 70% cocoa)
- 1/4 cup chopped almonds

Instructions:

1. Melt the dark chocolate in a microwave-safe bowl, stirring every 30 seconds until smooth.

2. Spread the melted chocolate on a parchment-lined baking sheet.

3. Sprinkle chopped almonds evenly over the chocolate.

4. Place in the refrigerator for about 30 minutes or until the chocolate hardens.

5. Break into pieces and enjoy the rich and crunchy dark chocolate bark

Vanilla Panna Cotta with Mixed Berries:

Ingredients:

- 1 cup unsweetened almond milk
- 1 teaspoon vanilla extract
- 1 tablespoon gelatin powder
- 1 tablespoon honey or sugar substitute (optional)

- Mixed berries for topping

Instructions:

1. Warm the almond milk and vanilla essence in a saucepan over medium heat until steaming.

2. Dissolve gelatin powder with 1/4 cup cold water in a separate basin.

3. Stir in the dissolved gelatin into the heated almond milk mixture until fully mixed.

4. Remove from the heat and set aside to cool somewhat.

5. If desired, add honey or a sugar alternative.

6. Refrigerate the mixture in serving glasses or ramekins for at least 4 hours, or until set.

7. Serve the cold panna cotta with mixed berries on top.

Banana ice Cream:

Ingredients:

- 2 ripe bananas, peeled and frozen
- 1 tablespoon unsweetened cocoa powder (optional)
- 1 tablespoon natural peanut butter (optional)

Instructions:

1. In a blender or food processor, combine frozen bananas.
2. Blend until the mixture is smooth and creamy.
3. Add cocoa powder and mix again for a chocolate taste.
4. Add peanut butter and mix until completely incorporated for a nutty twist.
5. Serve right away as a guilt-free ice cream substitute.

Baked Apple Chips:

Ingredients:

- 2 apples, cored and thinly sliced
- 1 teaspoon ground cinnamon

Instructions:

1. Preheat the oven to 200°F (95°C).
2. Place the apple slices on a parchment-lined baking sheet.
3. Sprinkle cinnamon over the apple slices.
4. Bake for 2-3 hours or until the chips are crisp.
5. Let them cool before enjoying these naturally sweet and crunchy treats.

Chia Seed Pudding with Berries:

Ingredients:

- 2 tablespoons chia seeds
- 1 cup unsweetened almond milk
- 1 tablespoon honey or sugar substitute (optional)

- Fresh berries for topping

Instructions:

1. Chia seeds and almond milk should be combined in a container or dish.
2. Stir well to avoid clumping.
3. Allow the mixture to settle for 5 minutes before stirring again.
4. Cover and place in the refrigerator for at least 2 hours or overnight.
5. If desired, sweeten with honey or a sugar alternative.
6. Before serving, sprinkle with fresh berries.

Baked Peaches with Cinnamon and Walnuts:

Ingredients:

- 2 ripe peaches, halved and pitted
- 1 tablespoon melted coconut oil or butter
- 1 teaspoon ground cinnamon

- 2 tablespoons chopped walnuts

- 1 teaspoon honey or sugar substitute (optional)

Instructions:

1. Preheat the oven to 375 degrees Fahrenheit (190 degrees Celsius).

2. Place the peach halves cut side up on a baking sheet.

3. Brush the peaches with the melted coconut oil or butter.

4. Sprinkle cinnamon and walnuts on top of each peach half.

5. If desired, drizzle with honey or sprinkle with a sugar alternative.

6. Bake the peaches for 15-20 minutes, or until soft.

7. Serve warm as a warm, naturally sweet dessert.

Yogurt Parfait with Fresh Fruit:

Ingredients:

- 1 cup Greek yogurt (plain or unsweetened)
- 1/4 cup mixed fresh berries (such as blueberries, strawberries, and raspberries)
- 1 tablespoon chopped nuts (such as almonds or walnuts)
- 1 teaspoon honey or sugar substitute (optional)

Instructions:

1. Layer Greek yogurt, fresh berries, and chopped almonds in a glass or dish.
2. If desired, drizzle with honey or sprinkle with a sugar alternative.
3. Rep the layers until all of the ingredients have been utilized.
4. Serve chilled as a light, protein-rich dessert.

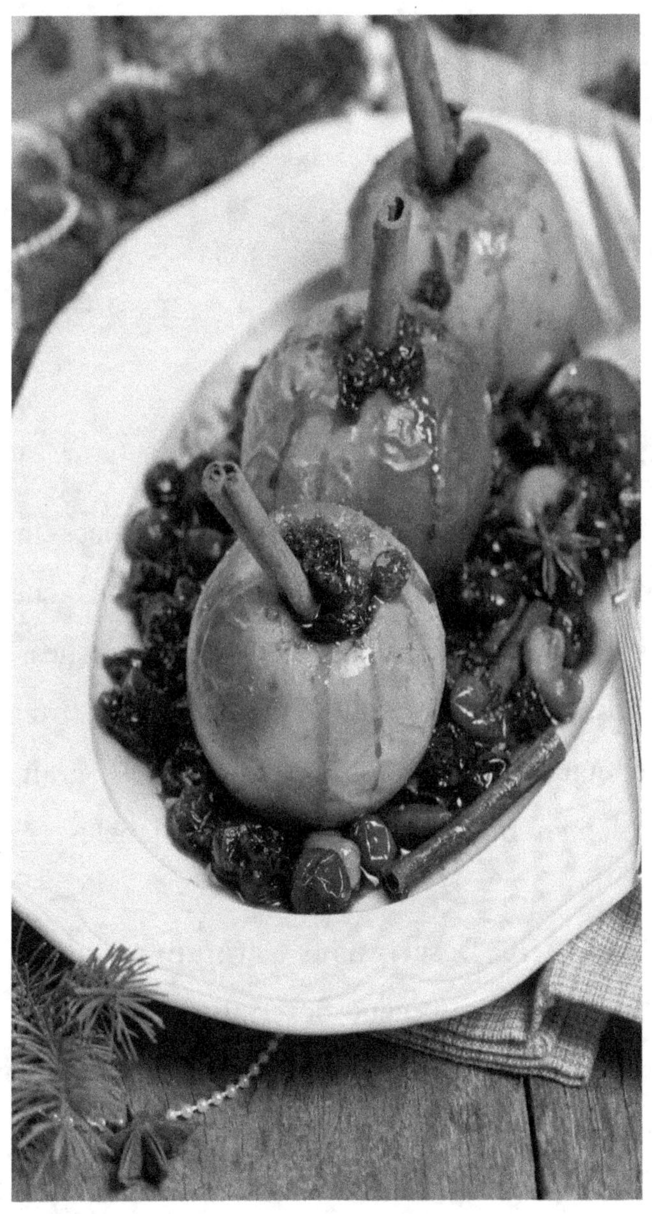

CHAPTER 7

TIPS AND TRICKS FOR DINNING OUT

Tips for ordering diabetes-Friendly meals at home

Choose Healthy Cuisine Options:

Look for restaurants or delivery services that offer a variety of healthy cuisine options, such as Mediterranean, Asian, or vegetarian dishes. These cuisines often incorporate fresh vegetables, lean proteins, and whole grains, which are beneficial for managing diabetes.

Read Menu Descriptions Carefully:

Pay attention to menu descriptions and choose dishes that are grilled, baked, steamed, or roasted instead of fried or breaded.

Look for keywords like "grilled," "broiled," "poached," "steamed," or "oven-roasted" to identify healthier cooking methods.

Opt for Lean Proteins:

Choose dishes that include lean protein sources such as skinless poultry, fish, seafood, or tofu. Avoid dishes with fatty cuts of meat or excessive amounts of processed meats.

Emphasize Non-Starchy Vegetables:

Prioritize dishes that contain a variety of non-starchy vegetables like broccoli, spinach, peppers, mushrooms, or zucchini.
These vegetables are low in carbohydrates and rich in fiber, vitamins, and minerals.

Be Mindful of Carbohydrates:

Pay attention to carbohydrate-containing ingredients like rice, pasta, bread, or potatoes in the dish.

Opt for whole grain options when available, or consider requesting smaller portions or substitutes like cauliflower rice or zucchini noodles.

Request Sauce and Dressing on the Side:

Ask for sauces, dressings, or gravies to be served on the side.

This way, you can control the amount you use, which helps manage added sugars, sodium, and unhealthy fats.

Customize Your Order:

Don't hesitate to request modifications to suit your dietary needs.

Ask for items to be prepared without added salt, sugar, or unhealthy oils, and request additional vegetables or a side salad instead of high-carb sides.

Pay Attention to Portion Sizes:

Be aware of portion sizes and consider sharing meals or requesting a smaller portion if available.

This can help control calorie intake and prevent overeating.

Hydrate with Water:

Instead of sugary drinks or sodas, opt for water or unsweetened beverages to stay hydrated and avoid unnecessary added sugars.

Plan Ahead:

If ordering from a delivery service, review the menu in advance to make informed choices.

Consider calling the restaurant directly to inquire about the ingredients or discuss any specific dietary needs or concerns.

Look for Nutrient-Dense Options:

Choose meals that are nutrient-dense and provide a balance of macronutrients (carbohydrates, protein, and fats) as well as essential vitamins and minerals.

Seek out meals that incorporate a variety of colorful vegetables, whole grains, and lean proteins.

Control Sodium Intake:

Ask for dishes with reduced sodium or request that salt be omitted during preparation.

Avoid meals that are heavily seasoned or contain high-sodium ingredients like processed meats, canned sauces, or condiments

Be Mindful of Hidden Sugars:

Check the ingredients and nutritional information to ensure that the meal does not contain hidden sugars or excessive amounts of added sugars.

Avoid meals that are heavily sweetened or include sugary sauces, dressings, or desserts.

Pay Attention to Fiber:

Choose meals that are rich in dietary fiber, which helps regulate blood sugar levels and promotes overall digestive health.

Look for dishes that include whole grains, legumes, and fiber-rich vegetables.

Keep Hydration in Mind:

Opt for meals that are accompanied by hydrating options like water, herbal tea, or sugar-free beverages.

Avoid meals that come with sugary drinks or high-calorie beverages.

Monitor Blood Sugar Levels:

Remember to monitor your blood sugar levels before and after meals, especially if you're trying a new dish or if it contains unfamiliar ingredients.

Keep a record of your blood sugar readings to identify any patterns or triggers.

Be Prepared with Healthy Snacks:

If the meal doesn't fully meet your nutritional needs, have some diabetes-friendly snacks on hand to supplement your meal.

Opt for snacks that are low in carbohydrates, such as nuts, seeds, or vegetable sticks with hummus.

Example of diabetes-Friendly restaurant meals

Grilled Chicken Breast with Steamed Vegetables:

Grilled chicken breast seasoned with herbs and served with a side of steamed broccoli, carrots, and green beans.

Request the chicken to be cooked without added sauces or marinades.

Salmon Salad with Olive Oil Dressing:

Grilled or baked salmon fillet served on a bed of mixed greens, cherry tomatoes, cucumbers, and red onions.

Dress the salad with a drizzle of olive oil and a squeeze of fresh lemon juice.

Vegetable Stir-Fry with Tofu:

Assorted vegetables such as bell peppers, broccoli, mushrooms, and snap peas stir-fried with tofu in a light soy sauce or garlic sauce.

Request the stir-fry to be prepared with minimal oil and ask for the sauce to be served on the side.

Baked Cod with Quinoa and Roasted Asparagus:

Baked cod fillet seasoned with lemon and herbs, served with a side of cooked quinoa and roasted asparagus spears.

Ensure the cod is not breaded or fried, and request minimal added oil or butter during preparation.

Grilled Shrimp Skewers with Brown Rice

Turkey or Chicken Lettuce Wraps:

Ground turkey or chicken cooked with herbs, spices, and vegetables, served with lettuce leaves for wrapping.

Ensure the filling is prepared without added sugars or high-sodium sauces.

Quinoa and Black Bean Bowl with Grilled Chicken:

A bowl of cooked quinoa and black beans topped with grilled chicken, diced tomatoes, avocado slices, and a sprinkle of fresh herbs.

Request the chicken to be grilled without excessive oil or added sauces.

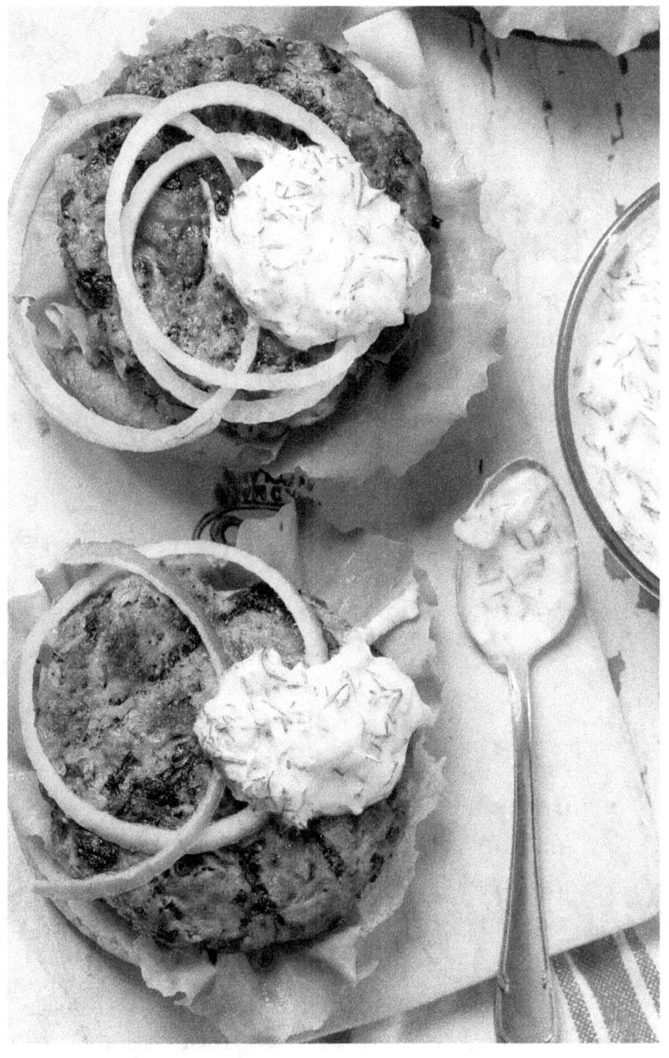

CONCLUSION

21-Day Diabetes Meal Plan (for individuals over 50's)

Day 1:

- **Breakfast**: Scrambled eggs with spinach and mushrooms, whole wheat toast.
- **Lunch**: Grilled chicken breast salad with mixed greens, cherry tomatoes, cucumbers, and balsamic vinaigrette.
- Snack: Greek yogurt with berries.
- **Dinner**: Baked salmon with roasted asparagus and quinoa.
- Dessert: Sugar-free Jello with whipped cream.

Day 2:

- **Breakfast**: Oatmeal topped with sliced almonds and blueberries.
- **Lunch**: Turkey or chicken lettuce wraps with avocado, bell peppers, and a side of cucumber salad.
- Snack: Celery sticks with almond butter.
- **Dinner**: Beef stir-fry with brown rice and stir-fried vegetables.
- Dessert: Sugar-free pudding cup.

Day 3:

- **Breakfast**: Vegetable omelette with feta cheese and whole grain toast.
- **Lunch**: Lentil soup with spinach and tomatoes, served with a side salad.
- Snack: Roasted chickpeas.
- **Dinner**: Baked cod with lemon and herbs, steamed broccoli, and cauliflower mash.
- Dessert: Dark chocolate square.

Day 4:

- **Breakfast**: Greek yogurt with sliced almonds and raspberries.
- **Lunch**: Grilled shrimp skewers with brown rice and steamed mixed vegetables.
- Snack: Baked Parmesan zucchini chips.
- **Dinner**: Stuffed bell peppers with lean ground beef and quinoa.
- Dessert: Berries with a dollop of whipped cream.

Day 5:

- **Breakfast**: Spinach and mushroom omelette with whole wheat toast.
- **Lunch**: Veggie and chickpea curry with cauliflower rice.
- Snack: Greek salad skewers.
- **Dinner**: Grilled chicken breast with quinoa and steamed asparagus.

- Dessert: Mini vegetable frittatas.

Day 6:

- **Breakfast**: Scrambled eggs with diced tomatoes and spinach, whole grain English muffin.
- **Lunch**: Baked chicken thighs with roasted sweet potatoes and a side of steamed green beans.
- Snack: Almond butter and apple slices.
- **Dinner**: Cauliflower fried rice with shrimp and mixed vegetables.
- Dessert: Sugar-free frozen yogurt with sliced strawberries.

Day 7:

- **Breakfast**: Overnight chia pudding with almond milk, topped with sliced bananas and chopped walnuts.
- **Lunch**: Turkey chili with kidney beans and diced vegetables, served with a side of mixed greens.
- Snack: Roasted edamame.
- **Dinner**: Grilled steak with roasted cauliflower mash and steamed broccoli.
- Dessert: Baked apple slices with cinnamon and a dollop of Greek yogurt.

Day 8:

- **Breakfast**: Veggie sticks with hummus and a hard-boiled egg.
- **Lunch**: Quinoa and black bean bowl with grilled chicken, cherry tomatoes, and avocado slices.
- Snack: Cucumber and tuna bites.
- **Dinner**: Baked salmon with lemon and dill, served with quinoa pilaf and roasted Brussels sprouts.
- Dessert: Mini caprese skewers with cherry tomatoes, mozzarella, and basil.

Day 9:

- **Breakfast**: Spinach and feta omelette with a side of whole grain toast.
- **Lunch**: Chicken or vegetable curry with cauliflower rice and a side of cucumber raita.
- Snack: Guacamole with baked tortilla chips.
- **Dinner**: Grilled chicken breast with steamed vegetables and a small serving of whole grain pasta.
- Dessert: Sugar-free lemon bars.

Day 10:

- **Breakfast**: Greek yogurt parfait with granola and mixed berries.
- **Lunch**: Lentil and vegetable stir-fry with brown rice.

- Snack: Smoked salmon roll-ups with cucumber and cream cheese.
- **Dinner**: Beef and vegetable stir-fry with quinoa.
- Dessert: Dark chocolate-covered strawberries.

Day 11:

- **Breakfast:** Oatmeal with sliced almonds, diced apples, and a sprinkle of cinnamon.
- **Lunch**: Greek salad with grilled chicken, feta cheese, Kalamata olives, and a drizzle of olive oil.
- Snack: Baked Parmesan zucchini chips.
- **Dinner**: Baked cod with lemon and herbs, served with roasted Brussels sprouts and quinoa.
- Dessert: Sugar-free mixed berry crumble.

Day 12:

- **Breakfast**: Veggie and cheese omelette with a side of whole wheat toast.
- **Lunch**: Spinach and mushroom quinoa bowl with roasted chickpeas.
- Snack: Celery sticks with peanut butter.
- **Dinner**: Stuffed bell peppers with lean ground turkey and quinoa.
- Dessert: Sugar-free vanilla pudding with fresh berries.

Day 13:

- **Breakfast**: Greek yogurt with sliced almonds and a drizzle of honey.
- **Lunch**: Lentil soup with spinach and tomatoes, served with a side salad.
- Snack: Roasted edamame.
- **Dinner**: Grilled chicken skewers with a side of roasted cauliflower mash and steamed asparagus.
- Dessert: Mini vegetable frittatas.

Day 14:

- **Breakfast**: Scrambled eggs with diced tomatoes and spinach, whole grain English muffin.
- **Lunch**: Baked chicken thighs with roasted sweet potatoes and a side of steamed green beans.
- Snack: Almond butter and apple slices.
- **Dinner**: Cauliflower fried rice with shrimp and mixed vegetables.
- Dessert: Sugar-free frozen yogurt with sliced strawberries.

Day 15:

- **Breakfast**: Chia seed pudding with almond milk and topped with fresh berries.
- **Lunch**: Turkey or chicken lettuce wraps with avocado, bell peppers, and a side of cucumber salad.

- Snack: Greek yogurt with a sprinkle of cinnamon.
- **Dinner**: Grilled salmon with roasted asparagus and quinoa.
- Dessert: Sugar-free strawberry cheesecake bites.

Day 16:

- **Breakfast**: Vegetable omelette with feta cheese and whole grain toast.
- **Lunch**: Lentil and vegetable stir-fry with brown rice.
- Snack: Roasted chickpeas.
- **Dinner**: Baked cod with lemon and herbs, steamed broccoli, and cauliflower mash.
- Dessert: Dark chocolate-covered almonds.

Day 17:

- **Breakfast**: Greek yogurt with sliced almonds and raspberries.
- **Lunch**: Grilled shrimp skewers with brown rice and steamed mixed vegetables.
- Snack: Baked Parmesan zucchini chips.
- **Dinner**: Stuffed bell peppers with lean ground beef and quinoa.
- Dessert: Mixed fruit salad with a drizzle of honey.

Day 18:

- **Breakfast**: Spinach and mushroom omelette with whole wheat toast.
- **Lunch**: Veggie and chickpea curry with cauliflower rice.
- Snack: Greek salad skewers.
- **Dinner**: Grilled chicken breast with quinoa and steamed asparagus.
- Dessert: Mini vegetable frittatas.

Day 19:

- **Breakfast**: Overnight oats with almond milk, topped with sliced bananas and chopped walnuts.
- **Lunch**: Turkey chili with kidney beans and diced vegetables, served with a side salad.
- Snack: Roasted edamame.
- **Dinner**: Grilled steak with roasted cauliflower mash and steamed broccoli.
- Dessert: Sugar-free blueberry muffins.

Day 20:

- **Breakfast**: Veggie sticks with hummus and a hard-boiled egg.
- **Lunch**: Quinoa and black bean bowl with grilled chicken, cherry tomatoes, and avocado slices.
- Snack: Cucumber and tuna bites.
- **Dinner**: Baked salmon with lemon and dill, served with quinoa pilaf and roasted Brussels sprouts.
- Dessert: Mixed berry smoothie.

Day 21:

- **Breakfast**: Spinach and feta omelette with a side of whole grain toast.
- **Lunch**: Chicken or vegetable curry with cauliflower rice and a side of cucumber raita.
- Snack: Guacamole with baked tortilla chips.
- **Dinner**: Grilled chicken breast with steamed vegetables and a small serving of whole grain pasta.
- Dessert: Sugar-free chocolate mousse.

BONUS: 10 JUICING RECIPES FOR DIABETES HEALTH

Green Delight:

- **Ingredients:** 2 cups spinach, 1 cucumber, 2 green apples, 1 lemon (peeled), 1-inch piece of ginger.
- **Directions:**Thoroughly wash the components. Remove the lemon peel and seeds. Combine all of the ingredients in a juicer and serve.

Beetroot Booster:

- **Ingredients**: 1 medium-sized beetroot, 2 carrots, 1 green apple, 1-inch piece of ginger.
- **Directions:** Peel and wash the beets, carrots, and apple. Reduce the size of the parts. Combine all of the ingredients in a juicer and serve.

Citrus Burst:

- **Ingredients:** 2 oranges, 1 grapefruit, 1 lemon (peeled), 1-inch piece of ginger.
- **Directions:** Peel the oranges, grapefruit, and lemon. Juice them together with the ginger. Serve chilled.

Berry Blast:

- **Ingredients:** 1 cup strawberries, 1 cup blueberries, 1 cup raspberries, 1 cup spinach.
- **Directions:** Wash all the ingredients. Juice the berries and spinach together. Stir well and serve over ice.

Cucumber Cooler:

- **Ingredients:** 1 cucumber, 2 celery stalks, 1 green apple, 1 lemon (peeled), a handful of fresh mint leaves.

- **Directions:** Wash the ingredients thoroughly. Cut them into smaller pieces. Juice everything together, including the mint leaves. Serve chilled

Pineapple Paradise:
- **Ingredients:** 2 cups fresh pineapple chunks, 1 cucumber, 1 green apple, 1 lime (peeled), a handful of fresh basil leaves.
- **Directions:** The ingredients should be washed and chopped into smaller pieces. Everything, including the basil leaves, should be juiced together. Serve with ice

Carrot Zinger:
- **Ingredients:** 4 medium-sized carrots, 1 orange, 1-inch piece of ginger.
- **Directions:** Peel and wash the carrots and orange. Juice them together with the ginger. Serve with a good stir.

Tropical Twist:
- **Ingredients:** 1 cup fresh mango chunks, 1 cup pineapple chunks, 1 banana, 1 cup spinach.

- **Directions:**All of the components should be washed. Mango, pineapple, banana, and spinach should all be juiced together. Chill before serving.

Kale Kick:

- **Ingredients:** 2 cups kale leaves, 1 green apple, 1 cucumber, 1 lemon (peeled), 1-inch piece of ginger.
- **Directions:**Thoroughly wash the components. Reduce the size of the parts. Combine everything in a juicer and serve.

Watermelon Refresher:
- **Ingredients:** 2 cups watermelon chunks, 1 lime (peeled), a handful of fresh mint leaves.
- **Directions:** Wash the watermelon and cut it into smaller pieces. Juice the watermelon, lime, and mint leaves together. Serve chilled.